Adverse Drug Reactions

Adverse Drug Reactions

Dinesh Badyal
MBBS MD (PGI)
Reader
Department of Pharmacology
Christian Medical College and Hospital
Ludhiana

R.S. Bhatia
MBBS DTM and H (Medicine)
DCAM; MNAS; FCCP; FICA (USA)
Consultant Chest Physician
Ludhiana

PEEPEE
PUBLISHERS AND DISTRIBUTORS (P) LTD.

Adverse Drug Reactions

Published by
Pawaninder P. Vij
Peepee Publishers and Distributors (P) Ltd.
Head Office: 160, Shakti Vihar, Pitam Pura
New Delhi-110 034
Corporate Office: 7/31, Ansari Road, Daryaganj
Post Box-7243, New Delhi 110002 (India)
Ph: 55195868, 23246245, 9811156083
e-mail: peepee160@yahoo.co.in
e-mail: peepee160@rediffmail.com
e-mail: peepee160@gmail.com
www.peepeepub.com

First Edition: **2006**

ISBN: 81-88867-88-8

Printed at
Lordson, C-5/19, Rana Pratap Bagh, Delhi-110 007

Preface

Medicine has changed, more so in the past three or four decades. The present day doctor has at his disposal a large number of potent drugs and hence it is very probable that these drugs can cause undesirable actions/ reactions, which have to be considered. In fact, these undesirable actions/reactions play a very important role in clinical practice today.

A number of reports of these unwanted and untoward reactions have appeared in literature. These publicized cases constitute merely the tip of an iceberg, a great many go unrecognized. Every one of us has to collaborate, to make the iceberg as small as possible, simultaneously keeping in mind that the iceberg will not melt completely by itself.

Before World War II it was said that a clinician who knows Syphilis well, knows more than ninety percent of medicine. All the pathological conditions known in medicine can be caused by *Treponema pallidum*. It would not be too far fetched to say that today a book on drugs induced diseases can take the place which used to be occupied earlier by clinical syphilogy. Drugs can also cause any disease listed in a textbook of medicine. There is one essential difference, drug induced diseases can be prevented if the physicians are aware of the causal connection.

A physician must be cautious in the administration of a drug. He must always ask himself whether the syndrome/disease with which, he is confronted could be caused by a drug prescribed to the patient. He must be well versed with the actions and reactions of drugs. The physician needs reliable and unprejudiced information to enable him to choose the best and least dangerous drug available, and a thorough knowledge about diseases caused by drugs.

The purpose of this book is to contribute to the prevention, recognition and treatment of adverse drug reactions.

Dinesh Badyal
R.S. Bhatia

Contents

CHAPTER ONE

Introduction

Human desire to take drugs for every disease is very strong. There is widespread use of drugs. More than 700 chemicals are used as drugs in the form of 2000 formulations. This is a well-known fact that drugs prescribed for diseases may themselves be the cause of adverse reactions, ranging from mere inconvenience to permanent disability and disease. During the past 25 years, 1 in 5 medicines were found to have serious side effects that were not recognized at the time of marketing.

At the beginning of 20th century syphilis was great mimic of systemic disorders. Later, tuberculosis took over this role. Both of these diseases have been tamed by chemotherapy and now "drugs" head the list of disease simulators. Drug induced diseases are gaining importance in this era of safe clinical practice and pharmacological advancement.

Adverse drug reactions (ADRs) have today assumed a differential diagnostic role in clinical medicine and are a cause of great concern. Earlier in 1961 it was toxicity of thalidomide, which led to its withdrawal. Thalidomide disaster caused birth of babies with defective limbs. Since the 'thalidomide' tragedy, there has been an increasing stress on identification of new ADRs and several methods have been developed for monitoring ADRs. However, this has not adequately prevented iatrogenic disasters. Recent withdrawal of rofecoxib has again highlighted the need to know about ADRs and their management.

Adverse Drug Reactions: A Growing Problem

During the last decade it has been demonstrated by a number of studies that morbidity and mortality due to ADRs is one of the major health problems which is beginning to be recognized by health professionals and the public. It was reported in the year 2000 that in USA 44,000 to 98,000 deaths occur annually from medical errors. Of this total, an estimated 7,000 deaths occurred due to ADRs. To put this in perspective, consider that 6,000 Americans die each year from workplace injuries. However, other studies conducted on hospitalized patient populations have placed much higher estimates on the overall incidence of serious ADRs. These studies estimate that 6.7% of hospitalized patients have a serious adverse drug reaction with a fatality rate of 0.32%. If these estimates are correct, then there are more than 2,216,000 serious ADRs in hospitalized patients, causing over 106,000 deaths annually. If this is true, then ADRs are the fourth leading cause of death in the USA after heart disease, cancer, and stroke and is ahead of pulmonary disease, diabetes, AIDS, pneumonia, accidents, and automobile deaths. The exact number of ADRs is not certain and is limited by methodological considerations. However, whatever the true number is, ADRs represent a significant public health problem that is preventable.

These ADRs result in the death of several thousands of patients each year and many more suffer from ADRs. Costs associated with drug-related morbidity and mortality were estimated at upto US $136 billion annually, which is more than the total cost of cardiovascular or diabetic care in the United States. In addition, 1 out of 5 injuries or deaths per year to hospitalized patients may be as a result of ADRs. Finally, a two-fold greater mean length of hospital stay, cost and mortality has been reported for hospitalized patients experiencing an ADR compared to a control group of patients without an adverse drug reaction.

Hospital admissions due to ADRs may be more than 10% of the total in some countries. For example, a 2004 study in the United Kingdom, carried out a prospective analysis of 18820 patients admitted into hospital over six months to assess the cause of admission. There were 1225 admissions related to an ADR, giving a prevalence of 6.5%, with the ADR directly leading to the admission in 80% of cases. The projected annual cost of such admissions to the National Health Service was £ 466 million (US $ 847 million).

According to a survey in 2001, the cost of detected drug-related morbidity and mortality in the United States exceeded US $177 billion in 2000, with hospital admissions accounting for about 70% of total costs. Since 1995, the costs associated with drug related problems have more than doubled. Approximately this is equal to the costs of medicines. Although the studies covered some four decades, there was no evidence of any systematic change in the rate of serious ADRs and the population studied was similar in most of the studies. Beside ADRs, medicine-related problems also include– drug abuse, misuse, poisoning, therapeutic failure and medication errors.

There is very limited information in the literature on ADRs in developing countries and countries in transition. However, it seems that the situation is worse rather than better. It is thought that adverse events in these countries are proportionately even higher than in wealthier regions. India has approximately 8 lakh practising doctors. Indian cities and villages are flooded with aggressive sale promotion by manufacturers. Use of over the counter (OTC) drugs and repeat prescription without adequate precautions are common. Many systems of medicine, Ayurvedic, Siddha, Unani and alternative system of medicine e.g. fish swallowing are common. Denial of adverse reaction by practitioners results in non-reporting of adverse reaction. Use of allopathic drugs by unqualified persons is also common. Aesthetic approach by qualified doctors cannot be ruled out at the same time. The coexisting factors are genetic predisposition, liver disorders, infections and aging population. Malnutrition may aggravate the situation. Widespread use of multiple drugs i.e. poly-pharmacy complicates and precipitates ADRs.

Are Drugs Safer Today?

It is said that a few people have to suffer or die to save others from toxic drugs. The following examples highlight this fact, as these drugs were introduced, they caused serious ADRs and then these drugs were withdrawn.

During 1960-1999 there were 121 safety related drug withdrawals worldwide. Market life was known for 87 of these drugs. Market life is less than 2 years for 31% products and less than 5 years for 50% products. Drug regulation process started in 1970s. Before marketing some data was required about drugs. During 1972-1994, 583 new active substances were approved, of these 59 were withdrawn later. During 1990-2001 in UK, 24 drugs were withdrawn due to safety reasons. In England and Wales the number of deaths related to ADRs has increased during last 10 years.

The rate of drug withdrawals has not changed over time. In the recent past critical opinions has been aired about the sale of many drugs from India that have been banned in other countries. World over nimesulide has been withdrawn, but continues to be sold in India. Nimesulide was discovered by an American company, but was never marketed in America. It has been banned by most of the countries including Bangladesh. Another drug that has been voluntarily withdrawn recently by the manufacturer from the world market was rofecoxib. The company's decision, which became effective from September 2004, was based on the three-year data from a prospective, randomized, placebo-controlled clinical trial. However, no alert was issued in India even after the media focused attention and pharmaceutical companies as usual, seem to be uninterested in voluntary recall. It has been withdrawn now in India. Now in public eye is phenylpropanolamine (PPA), a synthetic, sympathomimetic amine. It is almost ubiquitous in over-the-counter (OTC) cough/cold remedies and appetite suppressants. Reports link the use of these products to stroke. A survey conducted in the United States between 1994 and 1999 showed that women using PPA as appetite suppressant had higher incidence. The PPA-induced intraventricular hemorrhage has also been reported from India. Rightfully, the PPA has been banned in many developed countries but continues to be a common constituent of many formulations in India. Some companies have switched PPA but continue to retain its old brand name. The Family Welfare and Health Secretary, Government of India, has accepted that it has been alerted about PPA and are technically evaluating. In 2000, the US FDA issued a Public Health Advisory informing that it was taking steps to remove PPA from all drug products and has requested that all drug companies discontinue marketing products containing PPA. It warned of stroke risk associated with the PPA, and these drugs were removed from store shelves. In June 2001, Health Canada issued health advisory regarding PPA advising its citizens that after assessment of the safety of PPA, drug products containing PPA were being withdrawn from the market while we here in India still feel the need to evaluate it in 2006!

Rofecoxib is by no means the first drug to be summarily removed from the market. Cerivastatin and mibefradil suffered a similar fate, in both cases because of fatal toxicity due to interactions with other drugs. There are also many examples of new drugs, which have had significant safety warnings added to their product information within a few years of marketing. Table 1.1 gives some important drug withdrawals.

Why So Many Adverse Drug Reactions Occur?

There are so many reasons; few of the reasons are as follows:

Table 1.1. Withdrawn drugs and the cause of withdrawal

S.No.	*Drug*	*Reason*
1.	Triglitazone	Hepatic toxicity
2.	Rofecoxib	Thromboembolic episodes, MI, stroke
3.	Cisapride	Drug interactions
4.	Mibefradil	Drug interactions
5.	Nimesulide	Hepatic toxicity (still available in India)
6.	Bromfenac	Hepatic toxicity
7.	Alosetron	GI obstruction
8.	Phenylpro-panolamine	Stroke
9.	Cerivastatin	Rhabdomyolysis
10.	Encainide	Excessive mortality
11.	Terfenadine	Fatal cardiac arrhythmias
12.	Benoxaprofen	Liver necrosis
13.	Temafloxacin	Haemolytic anemia
14.	Rofecoxib	MI, stroke

- Availability of more drugs and more combinations of drugs used to treat patients than ever before. To exemplify this point, two-thirds of patient visits, result in a prescription. 2.8 billion outpatient prescriptions (10 per person in the United States) were filled in the year 2000.
- The rate of ADRs increases exponentially after a patient is on 4 or more medications.
- Wrong diagnosis of the patient's condition.
- Prescription of the wrong drug or wrong dosage of the right drug.
- Undetected medical, genetic or allergic condition in the patient which might cause a bad reaction to the drug.
- Self-medication (OTC drugs).
- Lack of adherence to the prescribed course of the drug.

This problem is also caused by a lack, in some countries, of legislation and proper drug regulations (including ADR reporting) a large number of substandard and counterfeit products circulating in their markets, a lack of independent information and the irrational use of drugs.

Efforts to reduce polypharmacy are important but for many patients, the number of medications cannot always be reduced without doing harm. That is why it is important to understand the basis for ADRs. This will allow us to make the most appropriate choices in prescribing and avoiding preventable ADRs.

Drugs undergo extensive experimentation in animals and humans, but still number of ADRs is not decreasing with new drugs. It is worth considering how well a drug's safety is defined prior to its approval and marketing. This will indicate how confident practitioners can be that a new drug's safety profile has been fully defined. Most new drugs are approved with an average of 1,500 patient exposures and usually for only relatively short periods of time. However, some drugs cause serious ADRs at very low frequencies and would require many more exposures to detect the reaction. For example, bromfenac was a non-steroidal anti-inflammatory agent (NSAID) that was removed from the market in 1998, less than 1 year after it was introduced. Bromfenac caused serious hepatotoxicity in only 1 in 20,000 patients taking the drug for longer than 10 days. To reliably detect the toxic effects of a drug with 1 in 20,000 adverse drug reaction frequency, the new drug studies would have to include 100,000 patients. A drug that is tested in a few thousand people may have an excellent safety profile in those few patients. However, within a short time after entering the market, the drug may be administered to several million patients, which actually happens. That means that ADRs which are not common, can only be detected after, not before, marketing.

If one case of hepatotoxicity is seen during pre-marketing testing, it can be difficult, if not impossible, to ascertain whether it was secondary to the drug or just the background rate of disease that is seen in the population. So, the safety profile for new drugs that come on the market is never totally defined because new drugs are studied only in relatively small and homogenous patient populations. The complete safety profile of a new drug will be defined only after it has been approved and is in use on the market. Hence, no drug is totally devoid of risk. However, a large proportion of ADRs of drugs are due to irrational use or human error and are therefore preventable.

However, it is important to remember that even when the above situations are carefully avoided, all medicines have side effects and some of those can be damaging. The effects of any medical intervention cannot be predicted with absolute certainty.

Adverse drug reactions can be minimized by an attending doctor only if he or she has update knowledge about ADRs. The knowledge to drug prescription, the monitoring of drug adverse reaction and to remain vigilant to recognize and record newer adverse reactions that has not been previously recognized. This is an important clinical issue. Those who want to think about it, and how it might be tackled, should read, digest and understand this careful and thoughtful piece of work.

CHAPTER TWO

Definitions, Mechanisms and Classification of ADRs

DEFINITIONS

Before defining ADR, let have a look at definition of the causative agent i.e. DRUG. WHO defines drug as "Any substance or product that is used or is intended to be used to modify or explore physiological systems or pathological states for the benefit of the recipient".

As per Drugs and Cosmetics Act (1940) in India drug is defined as "a substance for internal or external use of human beings or animals and all substances intended to be used for or in the diagnosis, treatment, mitigation or prevention of any disease or disorder in human beings or animals, including preparations applied on human body for the purpose of repelling insects like mosquitoes".

- Such substances (other than food) intend to affect the structure or any function of the human body or intended to be used for the destruction of insects which cause disease in human beings or animals, as may be specified from time to time by the Central Government by notification in the Official Gazette.
- All substances intended for use as components of a drug including empty gelatin capsules.
- Devices intended for internal or external use in the diagnosis, treatment, mitigation or prevention of disease or disorder in human beings or animals.

ADR is defined as harmful or seriously unpleasant effects occurring at doses intended for therapeutics, prophylactic or diagnostic effect and which call for reduction of dose or withdrawal of drug and/forecast hazard from future use. A large number of definitions of ADRs are available. US FDA defines ADR as "any experience associated with use of a drug whether or not considered drug related and includes any side effect, injury, toxicity, sensitivity reaction or significant failure of expected pharmacological action".

World health organization (WHO) defined ADRs as "a response to a drug that is noxious and unintended and that occurs at doses used in man for prophylaxis, diagnosis or therapy of the disease or modification of physiological function. This basic definition of WHO was given in 1972 and includes all doses prescribed clinically, but excludes accidental or deliberate overdose. The term "unexpected" was included under sub classification to facilitate understanding of the type of adverse reaction, which is most important to report to drug monitoring agencies.

Unexpected Adverse Reaction is Defined As

An adverse reaction, the nature or severity of which is not consistent with domestic labeling or market authorization or expected from characteristics of the drug.

These days a new term adverse event (AE) is also used. The use of term AE is more common during clinical trials. Some use this term interchangeably with "adverse reaction", but, as indicated, it is better reserved for clinical phenomena occurring during drug treatment where the possibility of a causal connection has not been considered.

Adverse Event/Adverse Experience is Defined As

Any untoward medical occurrence that may present during treatment with a pharmaceutical product but which does not necessarily have a causal relationship with this treatment. e.g. road accidents, falling from roof.

Most of us are very familiar with an older term "side effects". This term is broad enough to include both positive and negative effects of a drug apart from its main properties. Some use the term as synonymous with "adverse reaction", but the proposed definition will improve clarity of use of this term.

Side Effect is Defined As

Any unintended effect of a pharmaceutical product occurring at doses normally used in man which is related to the pharmacological properties of the drug.

There is another term used in ADRs. The term is Signal. This describes the first alert of a problem with a drug. By its nature a signal cannot be regarded as definitive but indicates the need for further enquiry or action. On the other hand it is prudent to avoid a multiplicity of signals based on single case reports since follow up of all such would be impractical and time consuming. The definition allows for some flexibility in approach to a signal based on the characteristics of individual problems.

Signal is Defined As

Reported information on a possible causal relationship between an adverse event and a drug, the relationship being unknown or incompletely documented previously. Usually more than a single report is required to generate a signal, depending upon the seriousness of the event and the quality of the information.

Categorization of ADRs

An ADR is categorized as serious if it:

1. Results in death.
2. Requires hospitalization.
3. Prolongation of current hospitalisation.
4. Causes a congenital anomaly.
5. Results in persistent and significant disability.
6. Requires intervention to prevent permanent impairment or damage.

7. Life threatening (is defined as an event in which the patient was at risk of death at the time of the reaction, which hypothetically might have caused death).

Intensity of ADRs can be:

1. *Mild:* An ADR, usually transient in nature and generally not interfering with normal activities.
2. *Moderate:* An ADR, which is sufficiently discomforting to interfere with normal activities.
3. *Severe:* An ADR, which is incapacitating and prevents normal activities.

Severe ADR does not mean that it is serious also. The term "severe" is not synonymous with serious. In the English language, "severe" is used to describe the intensity (severity) of a specific event (as in mild, moderate or severe); the event itself, however, may be of relatively minor medical significance (such as severe headache). Seriousness (not severity), which is based on patient/event outcome or action criteria serves as guide for defining regulatory reporting obligations.

The causal relationship of ADR to the drug can be classified as:

1. *Unlikely:* A clinical event, including laboratory test abnormality, with a temporal relationship to drug administration, which makes a causal relationship improbable. There is little evidence to suggest causal relationship (e.g. the reactions did not occur within a reasonable time after administration of drug) or there is another reasonable explanation for the reaction (e.g. the patient's clinical condition, other concomitant drugs). This definition is intended to be used when the exclusion of drug causality of a clinical reaction seems most plausible.
2. *Possible:* There is some evidence to suggest a causal relationship (e.g. reactions occurred within a reasonable time after administration of drug). However the influence of other factors may have contributed to the event (e.g. patient's clinical condition, concomitant drugs). Information on drug withdrawal may be lacking or unclear. This is the definition to be

used when drug causality is one of other possible causes for the described clinical event.

3. *Probable:* A clinical event, including laboratory test abnormality, with a reasonable time sequence to administration of the drug, unlikely to be attributed to concurrent disease or other concomitant drugs or chemicals, and which follows a clinically reasonable response on withdrawal (dechallenge). Rechallenge information is not required to fulfill this definition. This definition has less stringent wording than for "certain" and does not necessitate prior knowledge of drug characteristics or clinical adverse reaction phenomena. As stated no rechallenge information is needed, but confounding drug administration underlying disease must be absent.
4. *Certain:* There is clear evidence to suggest a causal relationship. The event occurred in a plausible time relationship to drug administration and which cannot be explained by concurrent disease or other drugs or chemicals. The response to withdrawal of the drug (dechallenge) should be clinically plausible. The event must be definitive pharmacological or phenomenological, using a satisfactory rechallenge procedure if necessary. It is recognized that this stringent definition will lead to very few reports meeting the criteria, but this is useful because of the special value of such reports. It is considered that time relationships between drug administration and the onset and course of the adverse event are important in causality analysis. So also is the consideration of confounding features, but due weight must be placed on the known pharmacological and other characteristics of the drug product being considered. Sometimes the clinical phenomena described will also be sufficiently specific to allow a confident causality assessment in the absence of confounding features and with appropriate time relationships, e.g. penicillin anaphylaxis.
5. *Unassessable:* There is insufficient or incomplete evidence to make a clinical judgment of the causal relationship. A report suggesting an adverse reaction, which cannot be judged because information is

insufficient or contradictory, and which cannot be supplemented or verified.

6. *Conditional/unclassified:* A clinical event, including laboratory test abnormality, reported as an adverse reaction, about which more data is essential for a proper assessment or the additional data are under examination.

Mechanisms of ADRs

A number of mechanisms are involved aetiology of typical ADRs: Drug reaction mechanisms may either be non-specific or specific to the patient. Some of these are as follows:

Non-specific reactions are:

- Overdose—excessive dosage leading to toxic effects, e.g. convulsions from overdose of lignocaine.
- Pharmacological side effects—side effects from pharmacological actions of the drug at therapeutic doses e.g. drowsiness from first generation H_1 antihistamines.
- Secondary drug effect—drug effect unrelated to primary pharmacologic action e.g. diuretic effect of theophylline.
- Drug interactions—where the action of a drug alters the efficacy or toxicity of another drug e.g. erythromycin increasing levels of theophylline through hepatic inhibition of metabolism.

Specific reactions are:

- Intolerance/idiosyncrasy—abnormal reactions to pharmacological effects, which may involve enzyme deficiencies e.g. hemolytic anaemia from G6PD deficiency with sulpha drugs.

Common Clinical Presentations of ADRs

Some of the common clinical presentation of ADRs are:

1. *Anaphylaxis*

   These are "Hypersensitivity Reactions"

   a. Immunologically mediated or anaphylactoid.

   b. Symptoms: Hives, laryngeal edema, nausea, vomiting, bronchospasm, hypotension.
   c. Seen with penicillin, aspirin, radiocontrast agents (anaphylactoid reaction).
2. *Cutaneous Reactions*
   a. Most common drug hypersensitivity.
   b. Idiosyncratic or immune complex.
   c. Hives common, treat with diphenhydramine or hydroxyzine.
   d. Maculopapular rash—Ampicillin with EBV infection, Sulfa drugs (especially in HIV).
   e. Erythema multiforme—Target-like (bull's-eye) raised maculopapular skin lesions.
   f. Stevens-Johnson syndrome—More serious ulcerations with mucosal eruptions.
   g. Stevens-Johnson is most commonly seen with sulfa drugs, allopurinol, anticonvulsants.
3. *Hepatitis*
   a. Usually with drugs metabolized by liver.
   b. Isoniazid—Slow acetylators.
   c. Halothane—Immunologically mediated.
   d. Alcohol ingestion aggravates most reactions.
   e. HMG-CoA Reductase Inhibitors.
   f. Antibiotics—Sulfa Drugs, Penicillins, Erythromycin, Tetracyclines.
   g. High doses of NSAIDs.
   h. Methotrexate.
   i. Alpha-methyldopa.
   j. Valproate, Dilantin, Carbamazepine.
   k. Nearly any drug can cause idiopathic hepatitis.
4. *Anemia*
   a. Hemolytic anemia is common.
   b. Non-immune mechanisms: e.g. G6PD deficiency (Antimalarials, Sulfa Drugs, Quinine).
   c. Immune Mediated (Coomb's Positive): such as Penicillin.
   d. Megaloblastic: Folate antagonists Methotrexate, Trimethoprim; also Zidovudine (AZT).
   e. Lupus-like Reactions—procainamide, quinidine, phenytoin, hydralazine.

5. *Neutropenia*
   a. Anti-neoplastic agents.
   b. Ganciclovir, sulfa drugs.
   c. Idiopathic: Chloramphenicol, ticlopidine, carbamazepine, felbamate, clozapine.
   d. Immunological: quinidine, heparin.
6. *Thrombocytopenia*
   a. Heparin, quinidine—immune mediated reactions.
   b. H-2 Antagonists (especially cimetidine)—direct toxicity.
7. *Hypersensitivity Vasculitis and Serum Sickness*
   a. Symptoms: arthralgias, rash, fever.
   b. Pulmonary inflammation with eosinophilia, macrophage activation, others may occur.
   c. Immune complex deposition may be important
   d. Seen most commonly with penicillin, aspirin, sulfonamides.

CLASSIFICATION OF ADRs

There are mainly two types of ADRs—A and B.

Type A (Augmented or Pharmacological) is the result of an augmented, or exaggerated pharmacological action of a drug, given in the therapeutic doses (Table 2.1). These are primarily dependent upon the intrinsic pharmacodynamic properties of the drug, often host-independent, dose-dependent and usually reproducible in animals. They are sometimes called predictable reactions, which include over dosage, side-effects, drug-caused disease and drug interactions. There reactions are common and avoidable. Examples include bradycardia with Beta-blocker, electrolyte disturbance with diuretics, hemorrhage with anticoagulants, Parkinsonism with antipsychotics, hypoglycemia with antidiabetics and galactorrhoea with alpha methyl dopa.

Type B (Bizarre or Idiosyncratic) reactions are totally bizarre or aberrant effects that are not to be expected from the known pharmacological effects of a drug when given in usual therapeutic doses and with no alteration in pharmacokinetic processes. They are "idiosyncratic", host-dependent, often apparently dose-independent and difficult to reproduce in animals. They are also classified as unpredictable, which include intolerance, idiosyncrasy and allergy. These reactions are responsible for most drug fatalities. Malignant hypertension with general anesthesia, acute porphyries, and drug induced haemolysis are some of the examples.

Table 2.1: Types of adverse drug reactions

	Type A	*Type B*
Drug Response	Augmented	Bizarre
Pharmacologically predictable	Yes	No
Possible to reproduce in animals	Usually possible	Difficult
Dose–dependent	Yes	No
Dependence on host	Often independent	Usually dependent
Incidence	High	Low
Morbidity	High	Low
Mortality	Low	High
Treatment	Dose adjustment	Stop

Type A reactions are more common, have high incidence and morbidity, but the mortality is generally low. By contrast, Type B reactions are usually severe and proportionately more often fatal. The incidence and morbidity of Type B ADRs are low and they are not observed during conventional pharmacological and toxicological screening programmes. They are usually detected only after a drug has been in general use for some time and this often results in the withdrawal of the drug e.g. zomepiruc-anaphylaxis mibefradil-drug interactions etc. Because of the severity, the Type B reactions have received exaggerated attention, however, there are no easy solutions to Type B reactions. Almost two-thirds of ADRs treated in hospitals are Type A and experts feel that these easily preventive ADRs should be given more attention. It is usually possible to make a distinction between Type A and B reactions, but in a few instances, both mechanisms may produce the same reaction, e.g. Chloramphenicol-induced agranulocytosis. The occurrence of both types of ADR depends on interplay between three factors—drug, patient and disease (Table 2.2), which are discussed below.

Table 2.2: Determinants of adverse drug reactions

1. Drug
i. Physicochemical properties ii. Pharmacokinetic characteristics iii. Dose iv. Route and rate of administration v. Other concomitant drugs vi. Inherent properties
2. Patient
i. Age ii. Sex iii. Pregnancy iv. Nutrition v. Allergic state vi. Genetic predisposition vii. Habits—alcohol, smoking
3. Disease
i. Underlying disease ii. Associated disease iii. Intercurrent illness
4. Prescriber

Type A Reactions

The factors involved in Type A reactions are those that modify therapeutic effects of the drug and they are divided into pharmaceutical, pharmacokinetic or pharmacodynamic causes.

Pharmaceutical Causes

Amongst the two factors—altered drug quantity or drug release, the latter is more common and important.

The release of active drug from a formulation depends on particle size, the nature and quantity of excipients used and the coating materials. The outbreak of phenytoin toxicity was due to a change of the excipient, which led to its increased bioavailability. Unexpectedly incidence of gastrointestinal haemorrhage due to rate-controlled indomethacin was due to irritant effects of a very high concentration of indomethacin at a localized area of intestinal mucosa. When taker full stomach, sustained release theophylline is rapidly absorbed, due to disruption of enteric coating in neutral pH, leading to dose-dumping and toxicity.

Pharmacokinetic Causes

Most Type A ADRs are due to a pharmacokinetic factor. Alteration in absorption, distribution, metabolism and elimination could lead to abnormally high concentrations of the drug at its site action and a correspondingly enhanced pharmacological effect.

Absorption: The rate and extent of drug absorption determining bioavailability can be affected by formulation, size and shape of tablets, excipients, GI mucosa and motility, hepatic first pass effect, other drug/s and food. Anticholinergic like properties reduces GI motility and enhances absorption e.g. digoxin. Food can increase the absorption e.g. propranalol, metoprolol and nifedipine and enhance their antihypertensive effects. Bioavailability of drug, with a large hepatic first like propranolol and nitroglycerine is increased in liver dysfunction.

Distribution: Drug distribution depends on hydro/ lipophilicity, regional blood flow plasma protein binding and tissue binding. In cardiac failure after haemorrhage, or after beta-blockade, liver flow is decreased and lignocaine clearance is reduced and high concentration may be observed after administration of large dose. Reduced plasma protein binding in hypoteinaemia results in enhanced response or toxicity of highly protein bound drugs like phenytoin, tolbutamide diazepam and diazoxide.

Metabolism: Drug metabolism is an important detoxification process in which lipid soluble compounds are converted to lipid-insoluble agents, which then undergo renal excretion. The metabolism predominantly occurs in liver in two phases. Phase I processes are oxidation, reduction or hydrolysis and Phase II process are glucuronidation, sulphation, methylation and acetylation. Reduced rates of metabolism will give rise to drug accumulation and increase the probability of Type A ADRs. Many common drugs e.g. tricyclic antidepressants, anticoagulants, anticonvulsants, benzodiazepines, antiarrhythmics and some beta blockers are metabolized by microsomal oxidation. As a result of individual variations in metabolism, patients receiving the same dose of 300 mg phenytoin develop plasma concentrations ranging from 4 mg/ml to 40 mg/ml and some will inevitably develop Type A reactions. In elderly, rates of microsomal oxidation of many drugs appear to decline, increasing the susceptibility to Type A reactions.

Some drugs show a genetic polymorphism for microsomal oxidation, e.g. debrisoquine. Poor metabolisers (PM) of debrisoquine are also PM for phenformin, some beta-blockers, phenacetin, flecainide and show impaired first pass metabolism thereby leading to increased systemic bioavailability and Type A reactions. Acetylation, which is the metabolic pathway for sulphonamides, dapsone, INH, hydralazine, procainamide etc. is also under genetic control. The incidence of rapid acetylators is highest amongst the Japanese and Eskimos (80-90%) and lowest in an African tribe (0.3%). Slow acetylators eliminate acetylated drugs much less rapidly than other people and are at greater risk from developing Type A reactions.

The active metabolites of drugs such as carbamazepine epoxide could also contribute to Type A actions of parent drug. Certain highly reactive metabolites, e.g. peroxides, epoxides, free radicals are responsible for cellular damage when the rate of their formation is enhanced or the rate of elimination is diminished, e.g. by depletion of glutathione. This is important in paracetamol poisoning.

Low-protein high-carbohydrate diet can inhibit metabolism of theophylline increasing the chances for toxicity. As liver is the seat of most of the metabolic processes, acute or chronic liver dysfunction produces impairment in a variety of pathways of drug metabolism affecting paracetamol, barbiturates, phenytoin and antipyrine and increases the potential for ADRs. In malnutrition there is impairment of metabolic pathways making the patients susceptible to toxicity.

Elimination: Reduced elimination leads to accumulation of a drug, with toxicity developing as a result of elevated plasma and tissue concentrations. Reduced glomerular filtration occurs in infancy and old age as well as in hypovolaemic shock and intrinsic renal diseases. Digoxin, aminoglycosides, ACE Inhibitors, flecainide, disopyramide and many cytotoxic agents are mainly eliminated by kidney and hence they are most likely to cause Type A ADRs. Vegetarian diet produces alkaline urine and high-protein diet produces acidic urine. This pH changes can explain some inter and intra individual sensitivities to drug effects.

Pharmacodynamic Causes

Pharmacodynamic depends, on dose-response relationship, drug receptor-binding and sensitivity, homeostatic mechanism and disease. The number and binding affinity of receptors affects target organ sensitivity. Reduced sensitivity of cardiac beta-receptors is known in the elderly. They are also more sensitive to effects of CNS drugs and warfarin. Thiazides have flat dose response in hypertension and increasing the dose of bendrofluazide from 2.5 to 10 mg increases the potential for electrolyte disturbances without improving the antihypertensive effect. The magnitude of drug effects depends upon homeostatic physiological controls.

Intercurrent disease can unmask pharmacological effects. GI haemorrhage due to aspirin-like drugs or corticosteroids is typical examples. Precipitation of neuromuscular blockade by streptomycin in myasthenia is wellknown. Bronchoconstriction with non-selective betablocker, like propranolol is not uncommon.

The basic mechanism of drug receptor antagonism or enzyme inhibition are not specific or totally selective for target tissues. Hence the same mechanism produces effects in target organs and unwanted effects in other organs. Aspirin, besides inhibiting synovial prostaglandins also inhibits gastric prostaglandins synthesis, which contributes to local ischemia and injury to gastric mucosa. Angiotensin converting enzyme (ACE) is important for renal function and ACE inhibitors are reported to cause renal failure in patients with declining renal function or unilateral renal artery stenosis or a single kidney.

Drugs like phenytoin with low or narrow therapeutic index are prone to produce Type A reactions if the dose increments are large and the clinical response is not carefully monitored.

Type B Reactions

Type B reactions, which are characterised by the existence of some qualitative difference either in the drug or in the patient or possibly in both, are classified as intolerance, idiosyncrasy and allergy. Intolerance occurs when a drug's qualitatively normal pharmacologic effect is quantitatively increased in a patient e.g. Salicylates induced tinnitus occurs in most individuals at high doses but in some even a single dose can produce the same effect. Idiosyncrasy is a qualitative abnormality not corresponding to a drug's usual, pharmacological action. Barbiturates may produce excitement in some patients. Allergic reaction is the result of an immune response produced by the formation of specific antibodies, of sensitized lymphocytes or both and, accounts for 3-25% of all ADRs. The causes of Type B reactions could be pharmaceutical, pharmacokinetic or may lie in a target organ response.

Pharmaceutical Causes

The potential sources are (1) decomposition of active substances (2) effects of additives, solubilizers, stabilisers, colourizer and excipients (3) by-products of the reactants of chemical synthesis. Paraldehyde older than 6 months decomposes to acetaldehyde and should be discarded. Propylene glycol, which is a solvent for phenytoin may be partially responsible for the hypotension following I.V. phenytoin. Recently, a new clinical entity called Eosinophilia-Myalgia has been described following the ingestion of L-tryptophan, which is probably due to a contaminant.

Pharmacokinetic Causes

Although theoretically possible, there are no documented Type B reactions attributable to abnormality in absorption and distribution. There is a need to conduct research in pharmacokinetic mechanisms of Type B reactions.

Pharmacodynamic Causes

Qualitative, differences in response to drugs may be considered as genetic, immunological or neoplastic and teratogenic.

Genetic Factors: These lead to "idiosyncrasy" and include various enzyme deficiencies, the best known being Glucose-6-Phosphate Dehydrogenase deficiency. The commonly involved drugs arc primaquine analgesics, chloramphenicol, sulphonamides and sulphones quinine and quinidine.

Apart from 2 main types of ADRs, the following types are also recognised:

Type C (Continuous) because of long term use of drugs e.g. tardive dyskinesia with antipsychotics.

Type D (Delayed) reactions which occur after months or years after using the drug e.g. carcinogenesis, teratogenicity.

Type E (Ending use) reactions are withdrawal is abrupt e.g. exacerbation of angina on abrupt withdrawal of beta-blockers.

Carcinogenicity: Several classes of drugs hormones, immunosuppressive drugs, and cytotoxic agents are known to induce malignancy. Daughters of mothers, who had been treated with stilboesterol in first trimester of pregnancy developed adenocarcinoma of vagina.

The carcinogenicity of cyclophosphamide, azanathioprine and chlorambucil is due to binding to DNA. The oncogenic effects of aflatoxin and benzpyrene are mediated by a formation of epoxides that bind to DNA. Sometimes the abnormal response to a drug may occur as a result of some potentially neoplastic tissue in the parent. A preneoplastic condition may be transformed into a frankly neoplastic state by administration of a drug e.g. oestrogen, which is given to treat some entirely unrelated condition. Underlying genetic abnormalities or surface phenotypes of the tumor being treated will influence susceptibility to the drug.

Teratogenicity: During pregnancy 45% of women may use at least one oral drug and the effects of drugs on fetus are a case of grave concern. Defects occur in about 2-3% of babies at births, of which 25% are of genetic origin and 65% are of unknown aetiology. Only 2-3% of these are linked to drug treatment. The effect of a particular drug on the developing fetus depends on the type of agent and the gestational age when it was taken. During the pre-embryonic phase (conception to 17 days) the result of an insult is either death or abortion or intact survival. The period of organogenesis, from 18-55 days after conception, is the period of maximum sensitivity and damage to differentiating tissues become irreparable. During the fetal phase from 56 days to term, the effect of drugs are usually limited to defects of growth and functional loss rather than gross structural abnormalities. The understanding of human teratogens remains poor but animal models provide some clues. Cleft palate induced in mice by glucocorticoids is believed to be due to cortisone tissue receptor complex altering RNA transcription and the production of lysosomal enzymes. It appears that there is a genetic and temporal susceptibility to a teratogenic which by specific processes causes a specific defect

Teratogenic Drugs

Drugs can affect fetus at various stages of development as follows:

1. During fertilization and implantation: from conception to 17 days.

2. Organogenesis: from 18-55 days. This is the most vulnerable period.
3. Growth and development: from 56 days onwards.

The following drugs can be harmful to fetus as per their risk:

A. Drugs which are Teratogenic in Human beings and Laboratory Animals

Thalidomide

The organs derived from the mesenchyme arc chiefly affected by thalidomide. In man malformations are more common in the upper extremities which maybe stunted to the state of stumps ending in deformed hands with the number of digits reduced to four. The lower limbs may also manifest reduction in the number of toes. All the joints are randomly aligned and the skeleton resembles that of a seal, hence this condition is called "phocomelia". In addition, syndactyly and triphalangia may also be observed. Other defects are: absence or dysplasia of the ear, cleft palate and abnormal dentition. Visceral malformations such as atresia of the oesophagus or duodenum, atresia of gall bladder, anorectal anomalies, tetralogy of Fallot and adrenal agenesis may also be often seen. Occasionally there may be microphthalmia and absence of semicircular canals. Among the laboratory animals, chick, rabbit and monkey are sensitive to the teratogenic actions of thalidomide and the anomalies observed are similar to those found in man.

Thalidomide has been remarketed for a number of intractable conditions. An written informed consent has to be taken from the patient to whom thalidomoide is prescribed.

Antiepileptics

Phenytoin has been reported to cause hair lip and cleft palate in babies born to epileptic mothers who received this drug during pregnancy. Diphenylhydantoin produce ectrodactyly, cleft lip, cleft palate, hydronephrosis and hydrocephalus in mice. Carbamazepine produces neural tube defects. Valproate produces spina bifida and other neural tube defects.

Steroids

Masculinisation of the female fetus has been attributed to administration of androgens during pregnancy. In addition to masculinisation of tube fetus, testosterone may produce permanent estrus in the rat at the time of adulthood. Diethylstilbestrol masculinises the fetus when injected into the pregnant woman. In the mouse and rat. the mouse and rat estradiol feminises the male and masculinises the female. Progesterone when given for maintaining pregnancy in women suffering from threatened abortions has been held responsible for masculinising effects upon the female fetuses. Masculinisation of the fetus in the rabbit has also been reported following administration of 17-ethinyltestosterone, a synthetic progesterone. Cortisone has been reported to give rise to birth defects in human beings such as cleft palate, gastroschisis, hydrocephalus and Fallot's tetralogy. In the mouse and rabbits cortisone produces palate and cardiac anomalies.

Antidiabetics

It seems that in human beings insulin is the least teratogenic of the known hypoglycemic agents. In the mouse insulin produces exophthalmia, umbilical hernia and fusion of the ribs. In the rabbit microphthalmia and spina bifida are commonly observed following insulin administration during pregnancy. Tolbutamide and chlorpropamide have been reported to be teratogenic in man. Tolbutamide produces absence of thumbs, syndactyly, malformed pinnae with meatal atresia, tetralogy of Fallot and multiple internal deformities. In the mouse spina bifida and anophthalmia are observed when tolbutamide was given.

Chemotherapeutic Agents

Sulfioxazole has been reported to be teratogenic in man. Sulfadimethoxypyrimidine when administered to pregnant rats and mice produces malformations of the teeth and skull in the offspring. Tetracyclines have been reported to be teratogenic in man. Among the experimental animals the chick is more sensitive to the teratogenic actions of tetracyclines. It produces discolored and deformed teeth and retards bone growth. It produced hand and foot defects in the fetus born to a patient receiving this drug. In the chickembryo and rabbit fetus, cyclophosphamide gives rise to malformations of the limbs. Busulfan when administered to a pregnant woman has been reported to produce hypoplasia of the ovaries and thyroid in the offspring. Busulfan is teratogenic and inhibits the male germinal line of the adult leading to sterility in the progeny.

Other Drugs

Warfarin produces nose, eye and hand defects. Lithium can produce fetal goiter and cardiac abnormalities. Indomethacin can lead to premature closure of ductus arteriosus. Isotretnoin causes craniofacial, heart and CNS defects.

B. Drugs Suspected to be Teratogenic in Human beings though Lacking Experimental Evidence

Trimethadione

It has been suspected to be teratogenic in humans. Mothers receiving this drug for treatment of epilepsy during pregnancy have given birth to offsprings with cleft palate, hydrocephalus and umbilical hernia. In laboratory animals no congenital anomalies could he produced with trimethadone.

Amitriptyline

Amitriptyline, an antidepressant related to imipramine has been also suspected to produce limb deformities in man.

Phenmetrazine

Phenmetrazine, an appetite suppressant when used by pregnant women has been reported to produce fetal malformation such as diaphragmatic hernia and limb deformities.

C. Drugs Proved to be Teratogenic Only in Experimental Animals

Chlorpromazine and promazine produce teratogenic effects in the rat. Pentobarbital produces birth defects of the skeleton in the rat. Sodium salicylate and phenylbutazone both produce teratogenic effects in the rat. Diphenhydramine and cyclizine are teratogenic in the mouse, rat and the rabbit. Nitrogen mustard in the rat causes deformed limbs, syndactyly andexencephaly and in the mouse atrophy of limbs, polydactyl, hydrocephalus and cleft palate. Chlorambucil It produces syndactyly and torsion of tail in the rat and cleft palate and umbilical hernia in the mouse. Actinomycin—D causes anencephaly, anophthalmia, microphthalmia, cleft palate and spina bifida in the rat and exencephaly and spina bifida in the rabbit.

In the chick, salts of barium and lead and sodium fluoride are teratogenic. Mercury salts produce anomalies in the mouse and chick. Several alkaloids used in therapeutics have been shown to be teratogenic in experimental animals, e.g. caffeine in the mouse, ergotamine and quinine in the rat and reserpine in the rabbit and the rat.

Utility of Know-how About ADR Mechanism

Simply the first and the foremost benefit are to develop antidote or specific treatment for specific drug reaction. Secondly it helps in the optimal dose of a particular drug. Also it helps in searching new dosage schedule for newer drugs. Chemical utility of drug dosage is best guided by Type A reactions. Studies for Type B reactions can make a path for better and safer drug developments. Use of RAST and bile salt sequestrants in rapidly growing serum thyroid levels shows the innovative role of applying adverse reaction to an advantage in therapeutic medicine.

Idiosyncratic reactions, unpredictable from knowledge of the basic pharmacology of the drug occur in a small percentage of the population, but are often serious and account for many drug induced deaths. Elucidating the cellular and chemical basis of idiosyncratic reactions is being investigated in recent years and methods are being developed to identify patients who have a genetically determined susceptibility. Such information can be used prospectively to avoid drug toxicities and in new drug development. The adverse reaction may be a function of the biology of the individual and chemistry of the drug. The hypersensitivity reactions associated with penicillin and cephalosporin are attributed to the presence of the strained beta lactam ring which is directly reactive to the nueleophilic group on protein producing a drug antigen. Genetic variation in drug biotransformation resulting in the formation of toxic metabolites and reduced clearance of such metabolites are probably responsible for toxicity to some drugs e.g. hepatotoxicity due to valproate. Some cellular detoxification reactions can be investigated using lymphocytes e.g., patients hypersensitive to phenytoin. These methods are now being applied to investigations of ADRs important to our population, e.g. hepatotoxicity to antitubercular drugs.

CHAPTER THREE

Drug Allergy

Drug allergy is a common ADR. Symptoms of drug allergy may include various reactions. Some of these reactions are:

1. *Acute Anaphylaxis:* This is the most feared response with its potential for sudden death characterized by shock and very low blood pressure due to systemic arteriolar dilation. Features include urticaria, angioedema, asthma, laryngeal oedema, hypotension, cardiac arrhythmias and gastrointestinal upset. The entire reaction is abrupt, explosive, but brief. Examples are bee sting and penicillin allergy. It is treated with epinephrine I.V., high dose fluids and vasopressor agents.
2. *Urticaria:* It is characterized by hives, wheel and flare response. Pruritis, often severe, is common. The reaction may be localized or systemic
3. *Serum sickness:* This reaction comprises of fever, urticaria, joint involvement and lymphadenopathy. It typically develops 1-3 weeks after drug therapy is commenced and may continue for weeks after the drug is stopped.
4. *Allergic rhinitis:* It is charaterised by rhinorrhea (excessive fluid and mucous secretion) because of obstruction and inflammation.
5. *Allergic asthma:* Due to eosinophilic infiltrate there is bronchospasm and also histamine induced hypertrophic smooth muscle in airways.
6. *Atopy:* It is constellation of atopic dermatitis (e.g. eczema), allergic rhinitis, allergic asthma. Patients usually have elevated serum IgE, typically to a

variety of antigens. There is increased risk of severe and fatal anaphylactic reactions.

7. *Anaphylactoid reactions:* These include radiocontrast media reactions, physical urticarias, aspirin sensitivity and exercise-induced asthma.
8. *Drug induced autoimmunity:* Some drugs are capable of inducing auto antibodies, which may not result in disease but can cause lupus erythematosus, hepatitis, etc. Numerous drugs induce immunological reactions in particular organs e.g. penicillin (acute urticaria), neomycin (contact dermatitis), methyldopa (haemolytic anaemia) and penicillamine (nephrotic syndrome).

Types of Reactions

Drug allergy is of four types:

Type I: Immediate Type (IgE Mediated): E.g. anaphylactic reaction to penicillins.

Type II: Antibody dependant cytotoxicity: Drug acts as a protein structure leading to formation of antibodies. e.g. penicillin induce hemolytic anemia.

Type III: Immune Complex Mediated (Complement mediated): Serum sickness, glomerulonephritis.

Type IV: Delayed Type: T Helper cell mediated.

Type I: Immediate Hypersensitivity (IgE Antibody Mediated) Reactions

These are classic allergic responses and occur in patients who have been previously exposed to the drug. It is mediated by drug specific IgE antibodies on the surfaces of mast cells or basophils, interacting with the drug to induce an array of chemical mediators. The response appears typically 30 minutes after drug administration, peaks in a few more minutes and subsides over a few hours. 'Anaphylactoid' reactions have similar clinical features to anaphylaxis, but they are not IgE-mediated. The time relationships may differ and prior drug exposure may be absent. The events are:

1. IgE antibodies bind mast cells, basophils, cross link IgE receptors causing degranulation.
2. Release of various mediators including histamine.
3. Leads to vascular leakage, especially venules.
4. The arteriolar dilation leads to hypotension.

Examples: Reactions due to poison ivy and anaphylactic reactions. Allergen immunotherapy can be beneficial by reducing specific IgE levels.

Type II: Antibody Mediated

IgG and IgM binding to fixed (not soluble) target antigens:

1. Initial sensitization, or cross reaction with infectious agent leading to antibody production.
2. Antibody binds to fixed antigen, attracts complement and Ig-Fc receptor bearing cells.
3. Complement (C')
   a. Human Antibody C' Activation IgM > IgG3 > IgG1 > IgG2 (IgG4 does not activate).
   b. However, IgG4 does stimulate C3a and C5a production, leading to neutrophil activation.
   c. IgG antibodies mediate platelet aggregation and neutrophil attraction.
   d. The pentameric nature of IgM Abs permit direct C' activation.
   e. However, unbound IgM cannot bind C1q due to steric effects (alleviated on Ag binding).
4. Platelet Aggregation
   a. Due to C3 attraction, platelet activating factor release.
   b. Leads to thrombus formation and vessel occlusion.
   c. Fibrinous inflammation.
5. Fc Receptor (FcR+) Positive Effector Cells:
   a. There are three main types of Fc Receptors for IgG (FcgRI, FcgRII, FcgRIII).
   b. IgG subclasses G1 and G3 bind FcR best, with G2 and G4 of lower affinity.
   c. Neutrophils, macrophages, B cells, and natural killer cells express FcgR.
   d. Binding of multiple Fc regions of antibodies to FcR signals these cells.

e. Both positive and negative signals have been identified in different systems.
f. In autoimmune (hypersensitivity) disease, effector cells mediate tissue destruction.

Examples of type II hypersensitivity include:

- Goodpasture's syndrome: Anti-glomerular basement membrane antibodies.
- Type I Diabetes Mellitus: Anti-ß-cell islet antibodies (Abs). Glucose intolerance and vasculopathy.
- Hashimoto's thyroiditis: Nonhyperthyroid, large goiter, anti-thyroglobulin Abs.
- Grave's disease: Autoimmune thyroiditis, with hyperthyroid. Anti-TSH-Receptor Abs.
- Myasthenia gravis: Anti-acetylcholine receptor Abs, leads to paralysis.
- Pemphigus vulgaris: Anti-epidermal cell adhesion molecule Abs causing skin lesions.
- Hyperacute graft rejection: Preformed anti-graft Abs in host.
- Autoimmune hemolytic anemia: Coombs' positive antibody mediated red cell destruction.
- Hemolytic transfusion reaction: From preformed anti-A or anti-B Abs (ABO grouping).
- Rheumatic fever: Due to antibodies to Streptococcal M proteins.
- Erythroblastosis fetalis: "Rh-Disease".

Type III: Immune Complex Mediated

1. IgG and IgM bind to circulating antigens (Ag) forming "immune" complexes (IC).
2. IC become extremely large mesh works with Ag bridges:
   a. Normal clearance is through C' binding (C3b) which reduces size of complex.
   b. C3b-IC then bind to complement receptor 1 (CR1), mainly on erythrocytes.
   c. C3b-IC bound to CR1 on erythrocytes are cleared in the spleen.
   d. Splenic uptake requires functional C2 protein.
   e. IC bind FcR as well on macrophages (mainly liver, some splenic) and can be cleared.

3. Failure of normal clearance mechanisms:
   a. May occur in persons with C' deficiency.
   b. May contribute to development of SLE and other immune complex disease.
   c. Large, uncleared IC are deposited on vessel walls, especially in the kidney.
   d. This leads to local C' and FcR+ cell activation and vessel damage.

Examples of Immune complex disease include:

- Systemic Lupus Erythematosis (SLE).
- Polyarteritis nodosa (PAN).
- Wegener's Granulomatosus.
- Bacterial Endocarditis, Henoch-Schönlein Purpura (Serum Sickness).

Type IV: Delayed Type Hypersensitivity (DTH)

1. Tissue damage within days to several weeks after the introduction of antigen.
2. Mediated by CD4+ T cells, sometimes called T-DTH.
3. Unclear if these cells differ from CD4+ T helper (TH) cells.
4. Requires intact antigen presenting cells, including Langerhan's cells of skin.
5. At least two exposures to the antigen, first for priming, second gives DTH.

Examples:

- Cutaneous sensitivity: reaction to poison ivy and poison sumac.
- Arthus reaction.
- First exposure: systemic I.V. injection of antigen:
  - Then give s.c. injection, and DTH reaction (wheel and flare) occurs in ~2 days.
- Allergic sensitivities: Cosmetics and detergents.
- Granulomatous disease.
- Sarcoidosis:
  - Tuberculin skin test: giant cell granulomatous formation.
  - Crohn's disease.
  - Spirochete diseases, especially Treponema pallidum.
- Deep Fungal Infections: e.g. histoplasmosis.

Special Considerations with Specific Drugs

Penicillin

Allergy to penicillin is the best-studied drug reaction. Anaphylaxis most commonly occurs between the ages of 20 and 49 years, but children and the elderly are not exempt. It is more likely to occur when the drug is given parenterally rather than orally. With the passage of time, 85% of patients 'lose' their hypersensitivity. Thus, allergy to penicillin (and presumably to other drugs) is not necessarily life-long. Penicillin allergic patients have 10 times the risk of other people of reacting adversely to other antibiotics.

Testing: BPO accounts for 95% of the metabolites of penicillin. Other metabolites, 'minor determinants', are also capable of inducing anaphylactic responses. In most of the places the skin test reagent benzylpenicilloyl (BPO)-polylysine is used for testing. A useful additional test reagent is freshly prepared benzylpenicillin (BP) (6000 U/mL), which may also detect patients allergic to minor determinants. A RAST for BPO is available, but a result is usually required quickly and a RAST result takes a few days. Testing with BPO alone fails to detect a significant number of patients at risk, but the addition of BP will improve the detection rate to 80%. This rate can be increased by additional testing with semisynthetic penicillins and particularly with preparations of their minor determinants. There is still a significantly high false negative group, so subsequent treatment with penicillin in test negative patients must be carried out with careful monitoring. To date, no skin test negative patient is known to have developed a severe reaction. That testing is useful has been indicated by studies of patients undergoing testing and subsequent treatment. In patients with positive tests, there is a high incidence of subsequent reactivity, those with negative tests have a very low incidence of reactions.

Ampicillin/Amoxicillin

Maculopapular rashes induced by ampicillin and amoxycillin are seen commonly in patients with infectious mononucleosis, cytomegalovirus and chronic lymphatic leukaemia. They typically develop 48 hours or more after drug administration and persist for a week or so. Unless the rash is clearly urticarial, it is unlikely to be IgE-mediated.

Cephalosporins

Cephalosporins and penicillin share the beta-lactam ring in their basic structure. However, clinical cross reactivity occurs in approximately 10% of patients. For patients allergic to penicillin, their chances of reacting to the cephalosporins appear no greater than those of reacting to other unrelated antibiotics.

Sulphonamides and Other Antibiotics

Despite the severity and frequency of allergic reactions, especially the trimethoprim/sulfamethoxazole combinations, there are no specific diagnostic reagents, which have been developed for commercial use to identify patients at risk of anaphylaxis. If desired, testing could be done with individual antibiotics as outlined above. There is a small potential for the Stevens-Johnson syndrome when testing for sulphonamides.

Multiple Drug Allergy

Many patients are being recognised as having allergic reactions to a number of antigenically unrelated drugs, antibiotics in particular. Indeed, one study of 312 penicillin allergic patients found that 21% of them experienced reactions to non-beta-lactam antibiotics. Clinical management is difficult, but should follow these basic principles:

- Preference should be given to antibiotics known to be tolerated.
- Patients who have reacted to one type of penicillin will not necessarily react to other types.
- Of the new classes of beta-lactams, the carbapenems (imipenem) cross react with the minor determinants of penicillin, whereas the monobactams (astreonam) do not.

- 'Third generation' cephalosporins have a lower incidence of allergic reactions than the 'first and second generation' drugs.

Drugs used in General Anaesthesia

Intradermal testing is highly accurate in identifying patients with a high risk of anaphylaxis to induction drugs (e.g. thiopentone) and to muscle relaxants (e.g. alcuronium and suxamethonium). Cross reactivity between muscle relaxants is often present.

Local Anaesthetics

These drugs are unlikely to cause IgE-mediated responses. Skin testing is probably warranted, with concentrations increasing to a typical therapeutic dose.

Radiographic Contrast Media (RCM)

Anaphylactoid reactions develop in 2-3% of patients. They may be more common with the use of ionic media. Most are mild (e.g. urticaria), but fatalities have been recorded. The aetiology is obscure, but IgE antibodies have never been demonstrated. Some features are:

- They often occur on the first exposure.
- Specific testing is useless.
- Patients with seafood allergy are at no greater risk.
- Pretreatment with antihistamines and steroids will reduce the risk of serious reactions.

Insulin

Bovine and pork insulins differ from human insulin in three and one amino acid sequences respectively. Adverse reactions to human (recombinant DNA) insulin are less likely to develop, but there have been isolated reports of patients allergic to animal insulins who have had cutaneous reactivity to the human insulin preparation.

There are two adverse immune responses: allergy and resistance. Large local swellings due to allergy are common and usually ease with continued treatment aided by antihistamines. Systemic reactions are rare and may require desensitisation. RAST and skin tests may be done. Insulin resistance is also rare and results from antiinsulin IgG antibodies which neutralise exogenous insulin.

Chymopapain

Anaphylaxis has occurred in 1% of patients treated by chemonucleolysis with chymopapain. As it often develops on first exposure, sensitisation may have resulted from meat tenderisers. Skin testing immediately before treatment is essential. The testing is done in sequence: prick tests of 1 mg/mL, 10 mg/mL and an intradermal test of 0.2 mL (100 micrograms/mL). If each is negative, the risk of anaphylaxis is minimal.

Streptokinase

Allergic reactions have been reported in up to 17% of patients treated with streptokinase. An intradermal test with 0.1 mL of 1000 IU/mL, if positive at 15 minutes, should detect those at risk of anaphylaxis.

Vaccines in Egg Sensitive Patients

Small amounts of egg protein may be found in vaccines for influenza, measles mumps rubella and yellow fever. Although allergic reactions in egg sensitive patients given these vaccines are rare, when in doubt, preliminary testing, firstly by prick and then intradermally, can be done.

Aspirin and Other Nonsteroidal Antiinflammatory Drugs (NSAIDs)

Anaphylactoid reactions to these drugs are not mediated through an immune mechanism. No objective testing is feasible and test dosing carries a high risk of severe reactions.

The factors, which predispose to drug allergy are: the drug, the patient and the disease for which the drug is given. Allergic "Urticaria" are caused by the interaction between drugs or their metabolites with various effector cells of immune system. As most drugs are small organic molecules (molecular weight < 1000 daltons), they are not readily recognised by immune effector cells and are called haptens. The drug or the drug metabolite combines with host proteins to form a drug protein or a drug metabolite-protein complex, which must have multiple antigenic sites to both stimulate initial sensitisation and subsequent allergic reactions. Initial exposure and sensitisation may induce production of drug specific or T-lymphocytes with drug-specific receptors on the cell surface. Re-administration of the drug at a later date may induce an allergic reaction in sensitized individual. The route of administration e.g. I.V. Determines the speed of adverse event. Penicillin, captopril and penicillamine, which are chemically reactive can react directly with tissue macromolecules. Drugs which are not intrinsically reactive are activated through metabolism, e.g. halothane. Once a drug protein complex has induced formation of specific antibodies or specific sensitized T lymphocytes, their subsequent interaction may cause tissue damage through four mechanisms of hypersensitivity described by Cell and Combs; immediate hypersensitivity, cytotoxic antibody, Immune-complex and cell-mediated hypersensitivity.

Many patients with glandular fever, viral infections or leukemia develop a skin rash with ampicillin. The rash appears to be due to an immunological abnormality induced by the diseases. When given prophylactically, antibiotics produce allergic reactions less frequently than when they are administered during infections. This is probably due to an adjuvant effect of bacterial endotoxin or increase in possible binding sites for hapten during infection. Some bacterial products may also potentiate the effects of chemical mediators like histamine.

Evaluation of Patients with Suspected Drug Allergy

History

This is the cardinal diagnostic tool. Key points include:

- Suspicion that an unexplained clinical event may be caused by a drug.

- Complete and accurate documentation of all drugs, including nonprescription ones, taken over the previous month.
- Temporal relationships between drug administration and the onset of symptoms or signs.
- Correlation of the clinical manifestations with known reactions induced by a particular drug.
- Previous tolerance of the drug (sensitisation).
- Prior history of a similar reaction to the same or cross reacting drug.

A few points should be stressed regarding the temporal relationships. It is virtually impossible to react allergically on the first exposure to a drug, never taken previously, unless the patient has had a crossreacting drug or unknown subclinical exposure to the drug or related compounds such as meat tenderisers (chymopapain) or quaternary ammonium compounds in cosmetics (muscle relaxants). Reactions occur within the first 7 days of treatment; rather, within 2-4 weeks. Further, if a drug has been taken continuously for a year or more, it is unlikely to cause a reaction. However, the classic IgE-mediated drug allergy typically appears after the first dose of a new course.

Patients who report an allergic response may have had an adverse reaction to the drug. Adverse reactions to drugs are common and drug allergy represents only about 10% of them. Certain clinical features help to distinguish allergy from other reactions:

- Only a small number of patients react in this way.
- Minute doses may trigger a response.
- The signs and symptoms are similar to those of allergic responses triggered by other substances (foods, animals, insect stings).
- They develop soon after the drug is started and resolve soon after it is withdrawn.
- They are quite different from the usual pharmacological actions of the drug.
- Specific tests may define the allergic response.

Testing is primarily restricted to the detection of drug specific IgE antibodies.

Tests

The tests which can be performed to assess drug allergy are as follows:
- In-vitro (RAST) testing.
- Skin testing.
- Challenge testing.

In vitro Testing

This has the advantage that adverse reactions to testing can be avoided. The most widely used is the radio-allergosorbent test (RAST), which measures circulating drug specific IgE antibodies. It is generally less specific and less sensitive than skin testing, thus limiting its clinical usefulness. These reactions involve immune (usually mast cell) activation, and have manifestations such as urticaria, angioedema or anaphylaxis. RASTs are only available for certain drugs such as:
- Beta-lactam antibiotics.
- Anaesthetic agents.
- Opioids such as morphine or codeine.

Skin Testing

Immediate type skin tests are the most rapid, convenient and reproducible method of detecting drug-specific IgE antibodies. They are most accurate in evaluating reactions induced by drugs, which are proteins (insulin, chymopapain, foreign antisera). Although skin tests for lower molecular weight compounds such as sulphonamides are of questionable value, exceptions include the major antigenic determinant of penicillin (benzyl-penicilloyl (BPO) compound) and some drugs used in general anaesthesia.

Skin tests are more sensitive than RASTs or in-vitro tests, and may be used for further testing in cases of suspected drug allergy where the RAST is negative or unavailable. However, like RASTs their usefulness is limited to IgE-mediated immediate hypersensitivity reactions. Skin tests may be made to confirm suspected allergies to drugs like penicillin or anaesthetic agents.

Prick testing should be done initially. The drug is appropriately diluted (e.g. 1:1000) with normal saline, a drop placed on the ventral surface of the forearm and the skin pricked through the drop. A positive response, read at 20 minutes, is a wheal 2 mm or greater than that of a normal saline control, and a surrounding flare. If negative, intradermal tests are done with serial dilutions. The forearm is injected intradermally with 0.05 mL of the lowest concentration (1:10 000 to 1:100 depending on the drug and the patient's history). A positive response at 20 minutes is a wheal and flare, with the wheal being larger than that raised by the initial injection and the normal saline control. If negative, the next (higher, usually 10-fold) concentration is injected.

Precautions

i. The tests are usually without risk, but anaphylaxis has occurred.
ii. They should be done by personnel familiar with the theory and practice of the procedure.
iii. The tester must be aware of appropriate starting dilutions as well as the concentrations likely to induce irritant (nonallergic) responses.
iv. False negative results may occur from:
   - Inappropriate test reagent.
   - Too short a time interval between the adverse reaction and test—at least two weeks is needed because a severe anaphylactic event temporarily depletes the circulating IgE antibodies and also the chemical mediators from the mast cells.
v. The patient may exhibit an anxiety or vasovagal response.
vi. Appropriate means of reversing a severe reaction must be readily available.
vii. Informed consent and accurate documentation are essential.

In vivo Testing (Challenge Testing)

Where there is suspicion of a drug allergy and a need to confirm the diagnosis in the setting of negative skin or *in vitro* tests, then controlled challenge with the drug is a useful diagnostic tool. Challenge testing, must be only performed by appropriately trained specialists, where resuscitation facilities are available. The initial dose is much lower, e.g. 1:100, than the usual therapeutic dose. Subsequent challenges are of higher concentrations than those used in the therapeutic technique of desensitisation. Frequency of dosing is determined by the type of the alleged drug reaction, at 30 minutes intervals for IgE-mediated reactions and 24-48 hours for a delayed response such as dermatitis.

General Management Principles

General management principles for patients with a history of allergy to a specific drug are:

- Obtain full clinical details of the reaction.
- If allergy is suspected, use an alternative, non-cross-reacting drug (available in most situations).
- If none appropriate, refer to someone competent in testing for drug allergy.
- Testing for suspected penicillin allergy should ideally employ different kinds of penicillins and cephalosporins as well.
- If tests are negative, give a test dose first where full resuscitation facilities are available.
- Treat minor allergic responses (especially rashes) symptomatically if continuation of the drug is considered essential, however, be vigilant for Stevens-Johnson syndrome (SJS) which is potentially fatal.
- Provide adequate follow up of patients.
- If the drug is required again, objective testing may be repeated.
- Know-how to treat anaphylaxis.
- If tests are positive, avoid the drug, however, desensitisation according to accepted protocols may be used as a last resort.

CHAPTER FOUR

Cutaneous ADRs

The skin and mucosae are the commonest organs for initial presentation of many serious adverse drug reactions. Cutaneous drug eruptions are one of the most common types of adverse reaction to drug therapy, with an overall incidence rate of 2–3% in hospitalized patients. Almost any drug can induce skin reactions and certain drug classes, such as non-steroidal anti-inflammatory drugs (NSAIDs), antibiotics and anti-epileptics, have drug eruption rates approaching 1-5%. Although most drug-related skin eruptions are not serious, some are severe and potentially life-threatening. Drug eruptions can also occur as part of a spectrum of multiorgan involvement, for example in drug-induced systemic lupus erythematosus (SLE).

Incidence is even much higher in the patients in Indian clinical practice but quite often not reported. Almost every physician has encountered maculopapular rash and fixed drug eruption (FDE) in day to day practice. Rarely, there can be delay in recognizing adverse drug reaction. The situation gets adversely affected in the presence of adverse drug interaction, leading to drug toxicity or treatment failure. Judicious management of these reactions requires a proper understanding of the various immunological phenomena in their patho-mechanism.

Factors, which may influence the occurrence of these drug reactions are:

1. *Age:* Immunological drug reactions are less common at the extremes of age, probably due to altered immunological responsiveness.

2. *Environmental factors:* Infectious agents, sun exposure, etc. may precipitate severe cutaneous ADRs.
3. *Genetic predisposition:* A genetic susceptibility in the causation of different cutaneous adverse drug reactions has been postulated. The association of Stevens-Johnson syndrome (SJS)—Toxic epidermal necrolysis (TEN) and drug hypersensitivity syndrome to specific HLA subtypes has been reported. Because of genetic basis, many drug reactions, especially to anticonvulsants, may occur within the family.
4. *Metabolic abnormality:* Severe cutaneous ADR are commoner in individuals with specific metabolic abnormalities. These involve defects in the different enzyme systems metabolizing the respective drugs, especially the phase II enzymes like glutathione-S transferase and epoxide hydroxylase. Slow acetylators are known to develop adverse drug reactions to sulphonamides. However, as about 50% of the population among any race are slow acetylators and serious drug reactions are rare events, other cofactors may be responsible for precipitating such occurrence in predisposed individuals. The metabolic defect involved in each drug reaction seems to be highly specific for individual drugs as cross reactivity is not seen between different groups like sulphonamides and anticonvulsants. In genetically predisposed individuals, the toxic metabolites generated from the defective metabolic pathway may bind covalently to keratinocyte proteins and these metabolite-protein adducts may trigger an immune response.

The pathogenesis of these eruptions may be either immunological or non-immunological. Macupapular rash tops the list of cutaneous adverse drug reactions followed by fixed drug eruption (FDE). Fixed drug eruption, however, was found to be absent in a series from USA, as compared to a series from North India where more than 1/3rd of cases of hypersensitive reactions to antimicrobials had fixed drug eruption.

Adverse cutaneous reactions may arise as a result of immunological or non-immunological mechanisms, where fixed drug eruption has been found to be associated with HLA B22 and CW1 antigens. Regional or racial variations have been documented in occurrence of FDE. This is further supported with example of FDE due to dapsone being the most common drug in a series from South Africa as compared to a Delhi series where dapsone induced FDE was almost absent although the drug had been in constant use. Maculopapular rash is mostly caused by amoxicillin, sulphonamides, fluoroquinolones and tetracyclines. In practice, ampicillin and amoxycillin are mostly responsible for urticaria rash, a delayed type of response has also been observed. Acneiform of cutaneous eruptions are rarely encountered to antimicrobials. The cutaneous reactions to sulphonamides and cotrimoxazole have not decreased in the recent years, perhaps, these are underreported. Even cutaneous reactions to trimethoprim have been observed. Out of 600 cases of typhoid, skin rash was seen in 5/50 cases treated with cotrimoxazole in a recent series. The occurrence SJS and TEN due to sulphonamides has been predominant apart from thiacetazone, ampicillin, and ciprofloxacin. There has been genetic predisposition due to presence of HLA A29, B12 and DR7. Frequency of cutaneous drug reactions to sulphonamides such as macupapular rash & TEN is higher in patients used in case of dual infection. Toxic epidermal necrolysis or Lyell Syndrome is often fatal. These patients are susceptible to severe skin infections including tetanus. While care needs to be exercised in using these drugs, early detection and management of severe reactions such as SJS and TEN is *very* important to avoid fatal complications.

Ciprofloxacin has been found to be responsible for almost 10% of adverse reactions in clinical practice, involving a variety of reactions including maculopapular rash, bullous drug eruptions, and FDE, possibly because of its escalated use. In the recent years cutaneous rash and photosensitization are reported with sparfloxacin also. Cutaneous adverse reactions to rifampicin have also been documented in clinical practice, so are the infrequent cutaneous hyper sensitivity reactions to erythromycin and gentamycin. Commonly used antibiotics responsible for cutaneous adverse drug reactions are listed in Tables 4.1 and 4.2. As the trend of using antibiotics is always changing, so is the change in the pattern of adverse reactions of skin in the successive years. This is also affected to some extent by the drugs being co-administered as they quite often modify the drug reactions as has been seen with fluoroquinolones.

Table 4.1: Antimicrobials commonly implicated in cutaneous adverse reactions

Cotrimoxazole
Ampicillin and amoxycillin
Fluoroquinolones
Aminoglycosides
Tetracyclines
Anti Tuberculosis drug

Table 4.2: Commonly encountered cutaneous adverse reactions

Maculopapular rash
Erythema multiformae and acnieform eruption
Bullous eruption
FDE
SJS and TEN

Although most drug-related skin eruptions are not serious, some are severe and potentially life-threatening. Serious reactions include angiooedema, erythroderma, Stevens–Johnson syndrome and toxic epidermal necrolysis. Occurrence of unusual and severe forms of adverse drug reactions has never been as devastating as it is today. Most of the cutaneous adverse drug reactions occur within 24 hours of drug administration. Fatal reactions are almost always unpredictable, due to the complex underlying immunological mechanisms.

Characteristics of severe cutaneous ADRs include, prior exposure to the drug is necessary for the sensitization to occur and such exposure is without any effect. Once sensitization occurs, the reaction may occur within minutes to seconds. The reaction does not simulate pharmacological actions of the drug. It may follow exposure to doses that are far below the therapeutic dose. It is reproducible on re-administration of the drug.

A cutaneous drug reaction should be suspected in any patient who develops a rash during a course of drug therapy. The reaction may be due to any medicine the patient is currently taking or has recently been exposed to, including prescribed and over-the-counter medicines, herbal or homeopathic preparations, vaccines or contrast media. Remember that the non-drug components of a medicine, i.e. the pharmaceutical excipients, may cause hypersensitivity reactions in some patients.

CHAPTER FIVE

Gastrointestinal ADRs

Since most drugs taken by humans are administered by oral route, it is be expected that these drugs may produce some adverse reactions in the gastrointestinal tract (GIT). The entire GIT from the oral cavity to the rectum is susceptible to drug side effects during passage of the drug, after its absorption or its secretion during enterohepatic circulation. Though most drugs are considered "safe" when taken in the right dosage and for specific conditions, they can on occasion produce side effects either as a hypersensitivity reaction or dose related. Non specific side effects on the GIT are common to many drugs such as anorexia, nausea, vomiting, abdominal discomfort or burning and alteration in bowel, frequency either constipation or diarrhea, but what really concerns the physicians, is the drug induced GI diseases.

The exact magnitude of drug related GI toxicity is however not known. In developing countries like India with availability of drugs without prescription, frequent use of drug combinations, simultaneous use of herbal medicines, poor-record keeping and high incidence of gut infections it may be difficult to assess the exact magnitude of their side effects on the GIT.

NSAIDs and GIT Injury

One of the most commonly consumed drugs are the group of non-steroidal anti-inflammatory drugs (NSAIDs). About 10-30% of patients consuming NSAIDS have GI disturbances. Only a few studies have evaluated the GI side effects of NSAIDs and other drugs prospectively. Non-Steroidal anti-inflammatory drugs (NSAIDs) are one of the most widely used over the counter (OTC) drugs world wide. Although the extent of their usage in the Indian population is not known, it is likely to be large. Their major usage is as casual prescription for their analgesic and antiinflammatory action and in rheumatology and orthopedic practice. Sufficient evidence is now available regarding the mechanism of development of mucosal damage due to these drugs and also about contributing risk factors and the role of the type, dose and duration of NSAID used in causing them.

Pathogenesis

NSAID related mucosal damage is very important and is essential multifactorial injury. NSAID ingestion leads to denudation of mucosal epithelial cells and increased anion exchange. This leads to decrease in transmucosal potential which allows the drug to enter the cell. With change in pH of the milieu, the NSAID accumulates inside the cell and result in local damage. These mechanisms, either dependent or independent of the cyclo-oxygenase pathway also involve attenuation of the phospholipid membrane and surface hydrophobicity of gastric mucosal layer. The local effects are mainly erosion and acute haemorrhage.

Similarly systemic effect of NSAIDs on GI mucosa include an increase or similar incidence of gastric ulcer with enteric or nonenteric coated NSAIDs and also occurrence of gastroduodenal ulcers during NSAIDs use as rectal suppositories or by the parenteral route.

Cyclo-Oxygenase Dependent Effects

Cyclo-oxygenase (COX) is an enzyme that exists in two forms e.g., COX. 1 and COX 2. COX 1 is present in most human tissue especially in GI mucus and platelets. It acts upon arachidonic acid in cells containing phospholipids in their wall, resulting in the formation of different types of prostaglandins (PGE_2, $PGF_2\alpha$) in humans. Prostaglandins (PGs) are crucial in maintaining mucosal integrity by various mechanisms e.g. maintenance of mucosal flow, stimulation of secretion of gastric mucus, maintaining mucosal bicarbonate content and prevention of disruption of gastric mucosal barrier. Older-generation NSAIDs (aspirin, ibuprofen, naproxen, ketorolac) are non-selective, whereas rofecoxib and celecoxib represent a group of selective or COX 2 inhibitors. COX inhibition by non specific NSAIDs which inhibit both COX 1 and COX 2, result in reduction of inflammation, pain, fever and similar effects of inflammation by causing PG inhibition but exposes gastric and duodenal mucosa (predominantly) to their toxic effects of uninhibited thromboxane effects. It was expected that COX 2 selective drugs will have less GI adverse effects, but long term studies do not support this hypothesis.

Other Mechanisms of NSAID Related GI Injury

There is poor correlation between gastric mucosal injury and degree of prostaglandin suppression. Other mechanisms which might play a role in gastric mucosal injury are:

1. NSAIDs augment pepsinogen secretion via a mechanism that is independent of PGs and is possibly via a calcium-dependent post-receptor mechanism.
2. There is direct inhibition of gastric mucosal blood flow leading to reduction in duodenal bicarbonate secretion and augmentation in gastric acid secretion.
3. Neutrophils also appear to contribute to NSAID related mucosal damage.

CLINICAL MANIFESTATIONS

Esophagus

Esophageal ulceration and strictures constitute the major adverse GI manifestations of NSAID intake. The exact mechanism of injury is not clear. Prolonged mucosal contact leading to mucosal disruption and exposure of esophageal mucosa to gastric acid injury appear to be responsible for esophageal mucosal injury. Strictures are less widely appreciated.

Stomach

Gastroduodenal lesions developing from NSAID use may not always be symptomatic. Endoscopic evidence of gastric ulcer occurs in 10% to 40% of individuals taking NSAIDs and duodenal ulcer is reported to occur in 4% to 15% in the first 3 months of use. Certain factors like prior peptic ulcer disease and NSAID-related GI complication, advanced age, concomitant use of glucocorticoids or anticoagulants, high or multiple doses of NSAIDs, ethanol use and presence of co-morbid illness are definitive risk factors. *Helicobacter pylori* and smoking are possible risk factors.

Small Intestine

NSAIDs cause small bowel mucosal damage in the form of strictures, diaphragms, enteropathy and serious complications such as perforation. The exact mechanism of small bowel damage is not known, but increased intestinal permeability, mucosal disruption and bacterial invasion causing blood and protein loss are some proposed mechanisms.

Autopsy studies showed the prevalence of small intestine ulcers to be 8.3% in the NSAID consuming population with rheumatoid arthritis vs. 0.6% in the control population. Diaphragms in the small intestine are less common, retrospective study showing their occurrence in up to 1.5% of users.

Small bowel enteropathy is used to describe diffuse intestinal inflammation and increased intestinal permeability. It includes a whole range of entities such is chronic GI blood loss, protein losing enteropathy, iron deficiency anemia, nutrients malabsorption, and fecal occult blood positivity. Blood loss is by far the commonest symptom. This part of the intestine is relatively inaccessible to endoscopy and radiological investigations are not very useful in diagnosis.

A majority of lesions are asymptomatic and so do not require treatment. Symptomatic strictures, diaphragms and perforatious require surgical correction. Stoppage of the drug is beneficial in patients with chronic GI blood loss when NSAIDs are suspected to be the cause. Protein loss can be prevented by the use of namebutone, coadministration of metronidazole as they reduce GI permeability changes. Later supports the theory of bacterial inflammation as a contributing factor to NSAID-related intestinal injury.

Colon

Colonic injury among NSAID users is less appreciated and diagnosed. Animal studies suggest fewer instances of colon lesions as compared to gastroduodenal ones. The right colon, especially the cecum is the prime site of ulceration. Diclofenac rectal suppositories have been reported to be linked with lower GI bleeding and colonic perforation. Colitis is frequently segmental, non-specific and occasionally may show features suggesting eosinophilic infiltration or collagenous changes.

Anorectal diseases are generally seen with local use in the form of suppositories and may result in symptoms such us proctalgia, tenesmus, or watery diarrhea. Local pathology may vary from proctitis to ulcers and anorectal strictures.

Patients with pre-existing colonic disease may have worsening of symptoms on NSAID intake. Both alterative colitis and diverticular diseases are known to exacerbate during NSAID use.

Discontinuation of offending drug results in recovery within 3 weeks. Balloon dilation is conventional modality to treat colonic strictures and surgery can be reserved for resistant cases.

Management of NSAID-related Gastroduodenal Injury

Various factors that influence treatment and prevention of gastro-duodenal ulcers in persons using NSAIDs include the type, dose and duration of drug used, concomitant drugs, age of patient and prior GI disease. Prostaglandin analogue have been studied for its efficacy to protect gastric mucosa from NSAID damage. Proton pump blockers are more effective in prevention of GI ulcers. The administration of a nitric oxide (NO) releasing derivative of naproxen to arthritic rats led significantly reduced incidence of GI mucosal events when compared to aspirin, naproxen and celecoxib. Aspirin not only reduced inflammatory mediators but also caused significantly higher GI injuries Celecoxib was able to reduce PGE2 and aspirin-triggered lipoxil. This is a pro-inflammatory mediator regulating neutrophils endothelium interface reactions. NO-releasing naproxen not only reduces pro-inflammatory mediators, it also reduces neutrophils adherence to endothelium, suggesting its potential as a safer analgesic with better safety profile. Prostaglandin analogue, misoprostol is the dug given for prevention and treatment of NSAID induces ulcers.

A human study supporting these findings has recently shown benefit of NO-releasing NSAIDs. COX-inhibiting nitric oxide donors (CINODs) are probably future NSAIDs that may provide adequate control of inflammation, fewer GI adverse effects and better profile for Neutrophils–endothelial reactions.

Guidelines for Appropriate Use of NSAIDs

Age above 65 prior GI events (complicated or uncomplicated) prior ingestion of any one of aspirin, steroid or warfarin; preclude the use of NSAIDs alone. These should always be given with proton pump inhibitor.

Misoprostol significantly reduces adverse effect of non-selective NSAIDs. H_2 receptor antagonists can be used to prevent or treat NSAIDs related GI injury.

The various parts of GIT may be also be affected by other drugs as follows:

Oral Cavity Lesions

Phenytoin and amlodipine can produce gum hyperplasia in some prolonged use. Tetracyclines used in infancy may produce yellowish discoloration of the teeth. Metronidazole and tinidazole are known to produce metallic taste, in the mouth as they are secreted in the saliva. Cytotoxic drugs, immunosuppressant and antimetabolites may produce severe oral liberation and *Candida* infection.

Esophageal Lesions

Drugs like tetracyclines, ascorbic acid, anticholinergics and NSAIDs can directly produce chemical injury to esophagus. A direct and prolonged contact of these drugs can produce a localized ulcer which is most often seen at T1 level in the upper esophagus. Dysphagia, odynophagia and bleeding may occur within 6-8 hours of drug ingestion. An acute presentation, history of drug ingestion and localized injury are diagnostic features of drug indeed esophagitis also known as "pill esophagitis". Esophagoscopy usually demonstrates single ulcer often circumscribed in the upper esophagus. Predisposing factors are:

- Patients with esophagical strictures.
- Motility disorders of the esophagus, extrinsic compression, consuming large size tablets, or
- Taking drug in lying down position without adequate water are particularly susceptible to such injuries.

Sucralfate slurry (one gram 4 times/day for 6-7 days) heals the ulcer in most cases.

Drugs like diazepam, nifedipine, theophylline and oral contraceptives reduce basal lower esophageal sphincteric pressure and also esophageal clearance from the lower one third leading to gastrophagial reflux disease. Long term use of these drugs and high doses may eventually lead to a break in the normal esophageal protective barrier and ulceration. Severe reflux, especially in children may present with bronchospasm. Treating these patients with theophylline only makes them worse. Radionuclide activity over the lungs a day after oral consumption of radiopharmaceuticals suggests reflux disease. Omitting the offending drug, elevating the head end of the bed by 6 inches, using H_2 receptor antagonists or proton pump inhibitor and a prokinetic drug usually controls reflux disease.

Antimetabolites, metronidazole, erythromycin and potassium chloride may produce severe vomiting which may lead to a Mallory Weiss tear and Hemet emesis. Most often bleeding is minor and requires no blood transfusion. Esophagoscopy reveals a linear tear in the mucosa on the esophageal side, cardiac side or at the gastro esophageal junction. Omitting the offending drug (if possible) and simultaneous use of prokinetic drugs like metoclopramide, domperidone or mosapride is useful.

Gastroduodenal Lesions

Aspirin and microfined aspirin is the most commonly and widely used NSAID. Both have been lesions shown to cause marked exfoliation of the surface epithelial cells of the human gastric mucosa by measuring the DNA content of the gastric aspirates. Aspirin breaks the gastric mucosal barrier to produce occult blood loss in the faeces. Besides aspirin, other NSAIDs, corticosteroids, potassium chloride and antimetabolites are also known to produce gastro duodenal erosions and ulcer related complications. Gastric damage can occur within minutes of aspirin ingestion causing acute mucosal injury. If further aspirin doses are given, most subjects will have erosions within 24 hours. Though the individual risk to develop serious ulcer complications with NSAIDs varies from 4 per 1,00,000 to 2 per 100 annually, it is not exactly known if an acute damage contributes to chronic ulceration and its complications in NSAID users. Retrospective case control studies have reported a five fold increase in the risk of developing gastric ulcer, three fold increase in gastric ulcer complications and increase in the risk of duodenal ulcer complications with the use of aspirin and other NSAIDs. However the relative risk of developing duodenal ulcer is not increased. NSAID related ulcer complications are commonly observed with old age, female sex, with high doses, in association with corticosteroids, with prior ulcer disease and occur during the first three months of treatment.

Unfortunately, two thirds of NSAID associated ulcer complications present without any premonitory symptoms. With the introduction of H_2 receptor antagonists, routine admissions for peptic ulcer disease and elective surgery for peptic ulcer have reduced significantly, but the incidence of ulcer complications remained unchanged or reduced only marginally.

The exact mechanism of NSAID induced damage is not well understood. Reduction in prostaglandins, reduced blood supply, reduced gastric mucus and bicarbonate secretion, impaired epithelial cell recreation and altered motility may individually or in combination lead to decreased cytoprotection and gastric duodenal injury. A recent study has shown that among patients taking NSAIDs, *H. pylori* infection was more commonly diagnosed in those who presented with gastropathy (37%) than those without lesions (11%). The frequency of *H. pylori* increased significantly with the severity of gastropathy (mucosal damage with or without bleeding lesions). It is suggested that *H. pylori* may be a risk factor of NSAID induced gastropathy..This appears to be one of the likely factors since NSAID induced gastroduodenal mucosal damage depends mainly on the presence of neutrophils which are present in large numbers in patients with chronic active gastritis caused by *H. pylori.* Thus anti *H. pylori* therapy may be considered as a prophylaxis against NSAID induced gastropathy. The "triple therapy" regimen consists of:

1. Antisecretory-omeprazole.
2. Antibiotic-clarithromycin.
3. Metronidazole/tinidazole.

All drugs are given twice a day for 2 weeks.

Until safer drugs are available, NSAIDs should be prescribed only when absolutely necessary and titrated individually for efficacy in the lowest doses. It has been shown that ibuprofen causes, significantly less, gastric mucosal damage than other NSAIDs and should thus be preferred over other NSAIDs. Patients with high risk of ulcer complications and in particular, elderly patients should best avoid NSAIDs or concomitantly use cytoprotectors like misoprostol (prostaglandin analogue) to reduce the incidence of gastro duodenal injury (bleeding/perforation).

Intestinal Lesions

Sustained release indomethacin used to protect gastro duodenal mucosa may produce ulceration with or without hemorrhage, perforation or strictures in the small and large intestine. Small bowel ulcers may heal with multiple areas of stenosis. This is known as "Diaphragm disease". Prolonged use of NSAIDs may lead to blood loss and increased absorption of luminal antigens. NSAIDs with prolonged enterohepatic circulation and sustained release preparations are associated with higher incidence of intestinal complications.

Collagenous colitis is an uncommon condition that affects the large bowel primarily in middle aged and elderly females and is characterised clinically by watery diarrhea and histologically by thickening of the subepithelial layer by a collagen band with chronic inflammation. Though its etiology remains unclear, a recent study has shown that NSAIDs such as aspirin, naproxen, ibuprofen and indomethacin may play a causative role. However the mechanism by which they cause these changes is not clear. Colitis may occur with mefenamic acid and piroxicam. Antibiotics like ampicillin, amoxycillin, clindamycin, lincomycin, cephalosporin, tetracycline, rifampicin and many others can lead to severe diarrhea.

The more severe form known as "pseudomembranous colitis" is produced by *clostridium difficile*. Colonoscopy shows characteristics psueudomembranes and congested ulcerated colonic mucosa. Prolonged use of NSAIDs may occasionally exacerbate ulcerative colitis or lead to ischemic colitis. Vasopressin, a commonly used drug for acute variceal bleeding and ergotamine used for acute episodes of migraine may produce intestinal ischemia. Development of intestinal infarction particularly in elderly patients carries a high mortality. If they are given antispasmodics for a long time can develop acquired megacolon or intestinal pseudo-obstruction. Prolonged use of irritant laxatives (anthracene group) can lead to mucosal pigmentation of the colon known as melanosis coli and may also develop a cathartic colon leading to lower abdominal pain and bloating sensation.

Pancreatic Lesions

Drugs are an important cause of acute idiopathic pancreatitis. Azathioprine, chlorthiazide, furosemide, sulfonamides, tetracyclines and estrogens are definitely reported to be responsible for acute pancreatitis in several case studies. Others like methyldopa, steroids, valproic acid and L-asperginase may also produce acute pancreatitis. Though the exact mechanism of drug induced injury is not known estrogens perhaps induce damage secondary to increased lipid levels.

Gall Bladder Lesions

Prolonged intralipid therapy in patients with massive intestinal resection, severe burns or malignancy leads to reduced gall bladder contractions and sludge formation, leading to symptomatic stone formation, pancreatitis or chronic cholecystitis. Long term use of the oral contraceptive pill reduces gall bladder contractility and doubles the risk of gall bladder disease. Cholesterol reducing drugs such as clofibrate increase biliary cholesterol excretion and make the bile lithogenic. Prolonged uses of cholestyramine reduce the bile acid pool and thus promote gall stone formation. NSAIDs may lead to biliary colic and cholestasis. Small doses of cholecystokinin or erythromycin may help prevent gall bladder sludge formation.

Factors Affecting Adverse Effects of Drugs on GI Tract

Risk factors which may predispose to developing adverse drug reaction are:

Age

Old patients who are more than 60 years age carry higher risk of gastric damage possibly due to lower cytoprotection combined with age related atrophic gastritis Hence these drug should be used with great caution in the elderly individuals. Incidence of ulcer complication is higher in females compared to male possibly due to higher consumption of NSAIDs.

Hepatic and Renal Function

Impaired hepatic or renal function may alter the metabolism and/or excretion of drugs and leads to increased drug levels for prolonged periods causing drug toxicity.

Pregnancy

Incidence of gastroesophageal reflux disease in pregnancy is further worsened by drug intake in the preexisting estrogen mediated reduction in basal lower esophageal sphincteric pressure and increased intra-abdominal pressure.

Gut Integrity

Gastric mucosa is highly susceptible to injury in patients with portal hypertension and uremia. Delayed gastric emptying in diabetic gastroparesis increases the risk of gastric irritant drugs.

Combination of Drugs

Steroids in combination with aspirin or other NSAIDs enhance gastric mucosal damage and may lead to ulcer perforation.

Drug Formulation

Enteric coated and slow release NSAIDs produce more small intestinal damage.

Dosage of Drug

Antacids, which besides neutralising gastric acid, also have a cytoprotective action, but if given in large quantities can produce diarrhoea (magnesium hydroxide) or constipation, (aluminium hydroxide). Thus, dosage should be titrated against the symptomatic need of the patient.

Golden Rules for Prevention of Adverse Reactions in GIT

Any drug may produce an unwanted or unexpected adverse reaction. Thus to prevent such reactions, it is imperative to follow some golden rules as follows:

1. Use only when there is a good indication.
2. Combinations should be avoided.
3. Use smallest effective dose and for a specified period.
4. Allergy and idiosyncrasy are important.

Greater awareness on the part of medical drug prescriptions require if GI disorders are to be prevented. All drugs should be used judiciously.

CHAPTER SIX

Hepatic ADRs

Recent data have shown that liver disease represents a larger percentage of adverse drug reactions than previously reported and that the incidence and severity of drug induced liver injury is underestimated among the general population. More than 1,000 drugs, ranging from NSAIDs to valproic acid, have been implicated in drug induced liver injuries, rendering the treatment of drug induced liver disease (DILD) an important but challenging task for health care professionals. Drug induced hepatic damage is the most frequent reason that new therapeutic agents are not approved by the FDA and is the most common adverse drug reaction leading to the withdrawal of a drug from the market. For example, ximelagatran, a promising oral anticoagulation medication, was denied FDA approval in September 2004 due to several cases of hepatotoxicity, including three liver injury associated deaths. Another drug troglitazone, a new antidiabetic was withdrawn after marketing due to hepatic toxicity. Nimesulide also can lead to hepatotoxicity and has been banned in a number of countries, but not in India.

Drug induced liver injury is the most frequent cause of acute liver failure and accounts for 15% of all liver transplantations in the U.S. In addition, this accounts for about 2% of hospitalized patients with jaundice and 25% of active chronic hepatitis. A population-based study in France from 1997 to 2000 reported that the incidence of drug induced hepatotoxicity was 13.9 cases per 100,000 patients per year, and the drugs most often responsible for hepatic damage were antimicrobials, psychotropic agents, lipid lowering agents and NSAIDs. These data demonstrated that observed incidence of DILD was 16 times greater than typically reported in postmarketing surveillance, indicating an underreporting of drug associated adverse events.

Drug induced liver disorders have a wide spectrum of all forms of liver disease (Table 6.1). Many present as subclinical liver disease and few present as fatal fulfillment hepatic failure. In fulminant drug induced hepatic failure, recovery is late and may need liver transplantation. A single drug can cause more than one type of liver damage.

Table 6.1: Presentation of drug induced liver Injury

Fatty liver
Hepatitis
Cholestatis
Mixed liver injury
Chronic hepatitis and cirrhosis
Hepatic granulomas
Veno-occlusive disease
Budd Chiari syndrome
Peliosis hepatitis
Neoplasm

Why Liver is Prone to Drug Induced Damage?

A principal function of the liver is the biotransformation of nonpolar substances to polar compounds that can be excreted in urine or bile. The enzymes that catalyze the biotransformation are usually found in hepatocytes and many of the substrates and the metabolites of biotransformation reactions are toxic. Subsequently, the liver is often the primary site of exposure to these toxins, and hepatic injury occurs frequently.

Drug Metabolism

Liver is the major sire of drug metabolism. It occurs in two phases.

Phase I or Non-synthetic reactions: These include oxidation reductions reactions, mostly catalyzed by the cytochrome P_{450} (CYP_{450}). These reactions tend to increase the polarity or water solubility of a molecule and therefore exposes a functional group on the drug as well as increases the potential for excretion.

Phase II or Synthetic reactions: These are conjugation reactions. Drug or product of drug produces in phase I reactions are conjugated with endogenous substances. Both phase I reaction and phase II reactions take place in mitochondria of hepatocytes (Tables 6.2 and 6.3). First phase metabolism, volume of distribution of drugs, half-life, protein binding and clearance of drugs affect the liver function.

Table 6.2: Drug metabolizing reaction

Phase 1	*Phase 2*
Non-synthetic	**Synthetic/Conjugation**
Oxidation-reduction (Cytochrome P450)	- Glucuronidation -Sulfation - Glutathione conjugation

Table 6.3: Drug metabolizing enzymes

Enzymes	*Subcellular Location*
Cytochrome P_{450}	Endoplasmic Reticulum
Glucuronyl Transferase	-do-
Sulfotransferase	Cytosol
Glutathione S.	Cytosol endoplasmic
Transferases	Reticulum

Although other metabolic pathways exist in drug metabolism, the primary metabolic pathways for most of the drugs involve CYP_{450} and subsequent esterification. Hepatocellular necrosis occurs through a process in which high-energy metabolites formed by CYP_{450} activation bind to cellular membranes or DNA and disrupt cell function. The best understood example of this process is acetaminophen-induced liver toxicity. Although safe in recommended doses, large amounts of acetaminophen cause cellular necrosis.

CYP_{450} enzymes consist of more than 30 different enzymes that demonstrate interindividual variation in activity and are susceptible to induction and inhibition by a number of substrates. This results in several drug interactions and an increased risk of drug induced liver injury. Individual variation in drug response may also be due to enzyme polymorphism, in which certain individuals lack the liver enzyme necessary for the metabolism of offending drugs that are associated with liver injury.

Alteration in immune response is another mechanism through which hepatocellular necrosis occurs. Studies suggest that a highly reactive intermediate formed by CYP_{450} metabolism covalently binds to the enzyme itself and evokes an immune response directed against newly formed metabolite-enzyme compounds. Inflammation and neutrophil-mediated hepatic injury may occur through another form of immune response involving cytokines (e.g. interferon, interleukin, tumor necrosis factor).

In phase II conjugation reactions, the binding of glutathione, glucuronate, or sulfate to metabolites produces nontoxic substances that are readily excreted through bile or urine. Glutathione conjugation is one of the most important defences against hepatocellular injury. Glutathione protects cellular enzymes and membranes from toxic metabolites. Inadequate stores of these binding substances can compromise efficient detoxification of reactive metabolites and the subsequent inability to detoxify toxic substances can result in liver injury. The rate-limiting factor for glutathione synthesis is the intracellular concentration of cysteine, which is often supplied in the form of N-acetylcysteine and replenishes glutathione in acute acetaminophen toxicity.

Factors Influencing Drug Metabolism

Development of hepatotoxicity depends on a balance between toxification and detoxification reactions. Several factors could influence this balance.

The nutritional status can influence expression of cytochrome and other enzymes and also availability of co-factors such as glutathione. Co-factor availability may be decreased under different situations. Ethanol can influence the availability of NADPH or UDP glucuronic and on large doses of determining acetaminophen may deplete glutathione.

An additional factor hepatotoxicity could be zonal distribution of enzymes. There is abundance of cytochrome P_{450} in zone III or glutathione in zone. Hence acetaminophen involves zone III and iron sulphate, phosphorus involve zone I in toxicity.

Classification of Hepatotoxic Drug Reactions

Drug injury to the liver could be of two broad types:

1. Predictable or intrinsic: occurring in many species on a dose.
2. Unpredictable idiosyncratic: occurring in a limited number, often with a small dose. They can produce pan lobular injury.

Intrinsic (predictable) and idiosyncratic (unpredictable) drug reactions can produce liver injury. Most drugs involved in hepatotoxicity belong to the idiosyncratic group. In most patients, intrinsic agents produce liver injury in a dose related manner when the toxic amount of drug is ingested. The hepatic injury can be due to direct hepatic necrosis, cholestatic injuries or both. Hepatotoxicity may be the result of the drug itself or more frequently, a result of the toxic effects of its metabolites. A number of drugs can lead to liver damage (Table 6.4). Among the listed drugs paracetamol (acetaminophen) is the most frequent hepatotoxic agent and can cause extensive hepatic necrosis with as little as 10 to 12 grams. Acetaminophen overdose is the most common cause of acute liver failure and death.

Table 6.4: Drugs that cause hepatitis

NSAIDs
• Salicylate • Paracetamol
Antibiotics
• Carbenicillin • Erythromycin estolate • Ketoconazole • Nitrofurantoin • Pyridium • Sulfonamide • Dapsone • Ethionamide • INH • Rifampicin
Cardiovascular drugs
• Acebutolol • Labetalol • Methyldopa • Quinidine • Verapamil • Felbamate • Valporate • Hydantoins
Immunosuppressant
• Methotrexate • Cyclophosphamide • Tacrine
Inhalation anesthetics
• Halothane • Methoxyflurane
Miscellaneous drugs
• Amiodarone • Lovastatin • Methimazole • Propylthiouracil

Idiosyncratic drug reactions occur in from one in 1,000 to one in 50,000 patients. These reactions are not due to the drug itself, since most people can tolerate the drug. Rather, unique patient characteristics, including genetic predisposition and a lack of enzymes required for the metabolism of certain drugs, may increase the risk of these adverse drug reactions. Idiosyncratic reactions occur in relatively small numbers. As a result, some drugs known to cause hepatic injury continue to be used, since the drug's benefit outweighs its risk. For example, isoniazid is implicated in about 15% to 20% of cases in which individuals develop increased transaminases after receiving the drug as a single agent for tuberculosis prophylaxis. Of these individuals, an estimated one in 1,000 may develop severe hepatic necrosis. NSAIDs, including cyclooxygenase-2 inhibitors, are also commonly associated with idiosyncratic liver injury.

Most idiosyncratic drug reactions are caused by hypersensitivity reactions and can result in damage to hepatocytes in the liver. The hepatic injury occurs within one to five weeks after initiation of drug therapy and is often accompanied by systemic characteristics of allergic drug reactions, such as rash and fever. Signs of hepatic injury reappear with subsequent administration of the same drug with only one or two doses. Examples of agents in which idiosyncratic drug reactions through hypersensitivity mechanism can occur include methyldopa, phenytoin, chlorpromazine and erythromycin (Table 6.5). Idiosyncratic drug reactions can also be caused by toxic drug metabolites. This form of drug reaction usually develops one week to 12 months after initiation of drug therapy and is usually not accompanied by systemic features of allergic reaction. Since the adverse effect is presumed to be the result of an accumulation of toxic metabolites, rechallenge requires administration of the drug that lasts from days to weeks for reproduction of the hepatic injury.

Histological Features Suggestive of Drug Hepatitis

Certain features are quite suggestive, though not pathogenic of drug hepatitis:

1. Disproportionately severe necrosis in comparison to patients.
2. Fatty change with acute hepatitis.

Table 6.5: Idiosyncratic drug induced liver damage

Drugs	*Forms of liver damage*
Isoniazid, trazodone, nefazodone, diclofenac, lovastatin	Hepatocellular necrosis
Estrogens, chlorpromazine, erythromycin	Cholestasis
Phenytoin, sulfamethoxazole	Immunoallergic reaction
Diltiazem, sulfonamides	Granulomatous hepatisis
Didanosine, valproic acid	Acute steatosis
Minocycline, nitrofurantoin	Autoimmune hepatitis
Methotrexate	Fibrosis
OCs, anabolic steroids	Tumours
Carbamazepine, cyclosporine	Mixed hepatocellular/ cholestatic injury

3. Non-caseating granulomas.
4. Bile duct damage.
5. Eosinophilic infiltrate.
6. Zonality i.e. sharp demarcation between the necrotic and non-necrotic parenchyma.

Liver cell necrosis or degeneration is the primary event, occurring acutely or chronically, the appearances could resemble sporty necrosis. This resembles acute vital hepatitis lobular disarray, diffuse ballooning of hepatocytes, and formation of acidophilic bodies. There is also infiltration of parenchyma mononuclear cells, plasma cells, etc. Examples are isoniazid, halothane, methyl dopa and phenylbutazone. Eosinophilia may be prominent with some drugs such as erythromycin estolate. The changes may resemble zonal necrosis. Typically involves zone III dropout of hepatocytes accumulation of PAS-positive ceroid filled kupffer cells and an "open" appearing reticulin around the central vein are characteristic. Examples are acetaminophen and carbon tetrachloride. The less common zone I necrosis (periportal) in seen with ferrous sulfate, phosphorus and cocaine. There may be massive hepatic necrosis. Agents causing spotty necrosis could also cause more severe injury, such as isoniazid and halothane. There is a collapse of reticulin framework with massive loss of hepatocytes. Proliferating bile ductules in periportal region (neocholangiates) are prominent.

Clinical Spectrum of Drug Induced Liver Disease

Most drugs associated with liver injury involve direct hepatocyte necrosis. However, some drugs cause cholestasis without significant hepatocyte damage or cause mixed injury, in which both hepatocellular and cholestatic damage occur. While in many drugs any of these three patterns may occur, most agents have a unique pattern of hepatotoxicity in the time of onset, frequency and type of hepatic injury observed. In addition, several other types of injury including steatosis, fibrosis and immunologic damage can occur with drug use. Various clinical presentations are:

Acute hepatocellular injury: Acute hepatic injury due to drugs may be hepatocellular, cholestatic, or a combination of the two. Hepatocellular reactions are the most common types of DILD and represent up to 90% of cases. Drug induced hepatocellular injury includes hepatic necrosis and steatosis, which can affect significant portions of the liver. Agents reported to cause hepatocellular necrosis include acetaminophen, methyldopa, valproic acid, trazodone, nefazodone, venlafaxine and lovastatin. Nefazodone was removed from the European market after numerous cases of hepatotoxicity, including fulminant liver failure and subsequent liver transplantation, was reported.

The injury is characterized by marked elevations (eight to 500 times the upper normal limit) in ALT and AST with variable elevation in bilirubin. Alkaline phosphatase value remains normal or only slightly elevated. These biochemical patterns resemble those of acute viral hepatitis and are often referred to as toxic hepatitis. The AST-to-ALT ratio is important in assessing hepatic injury from drugs. In alcoholic liver disease, including severe cases, the AST is always two to three times higher than the ALT but remains less than 300 IU, while the ALT is almost always less than 100 IU. In contrast, with most drugs causing acute hepatocellular necrosis, upper limits of these enzymes do not exist. Immense elevations in hepatic enzymes (5,000 to 10,000 IU) are most likely to be associated with acetaminophen or other chemical toxins and are unusual with other causes of liver disease, including acute viral hepatitis.

Clinical features of acute hepatocellular necrosis include fatigue, anorexia, nausea and jaundice. When hepatocellular necrosis is accompanied by jaundice, prognosis is remarkably worse, with reported fatality rates of 10% or greater. As hepatocellular necrosis progresses, clinical characteristics of acute liver failure such as jaundice, coagulopathy, ascites, hepatic encephalopathy and death may occur. Several other drugs are implicated in acute fulminant liver failure through the hepatocellular necrosis process as shown in Table 6.6.

Table 6.6: Drugs causing hepatocellular necrosis

Drug Group	*Drugs*
Antibiotics	Sulfonamides, Ketoconazole, Isoniazid, Rifampicin
Antiepileptics	Phenytoin, Carbamazepine, Felbamate
Analgesics	Paracetamol, Diclofenac, Bromfenac
Miscellaneous	Disulfiram, Propylthiouracil, Labetalol

Steatosis, another type of acute drug induced liver toxicity, is a condition in which the hepatocytes are filled with droplets of fat and can be present in a microvesicular or macrovesicular pattern. In cases of acute steatosis associated with drug use, a microvesicular pattern is present, in which hepatocytes contain numerous small fat vesicles distributed uniformly throughout the cytoplasm without displacing the nucleus. Acute steatosis due to drugs can cause enlargement of the liver and may also result in irreversible cell damage. Results of liver function tests may remain normal or elevated, although not as high as those reported with hepatocellular necrosis. Drugs associated with acute steatosis include valproic acid, tetracycline and aspirin. This form of drug-induced hepatitis is often asymptomatic and manifestations of clinical features such as malaise, diarrhea, fever, jaundice, ascites or edema indicate irreversible damage and poor prognosis.

Acute cholestatic injury: Cholestasis is a condition in which reduced secretion or obstruction of the biliary tree results in a reduction of bile flow. Cholestasis is characterized by elevations in alkaline phosphatase, gamma glutamyltranspeptidase and other indicators of bile duct injury. In most cases of drug associated cholestasis, symptoms of acute liver disease subside once the offending agent is withdrawn. Clinical manifestations include jaundice, pruritis, anorexia, malaise, pale stools, dark urine and fatigue. Amoxicillin/clavulanate is one of the most frequent causes of acute cholestatic injury that can resemble biliary obstruction. Other drugs associated with acute cholestasis include chlorpromazine, anabolic steroids and oral contraceptives (Table 6.7). Drug-induced cholestasis requires a longer time to resolve than hepatocellular drug reactions but usually has a good prognosis, with jaundice resolving within several months.

Table 6.7: Drugs causing cholestasis

Allopurinol
Amitriptyline
Azathioprine
Captopril
Carbamazepine
Chlordiazepoxide
Cyclosporine
Diazepam
Erythromycin
Gold salts
Haloperidol
Penicillamine
Phenytoin
Tolbutamide
Anabolic steroids
Androgens Estrogens
Phenytoin

Acute mixed injury: (Table 6.8) Drug induced injury in mixed form can be either primarily hepatocellular with cholestatic features or primarily cholestatic with characteristics of hepatocellular necrosis. With this injury, AST and ALT levels are elevated, usually more than eight times the upper normal limit. Alkaline phosphatase also increases to more than three times the upper normal limit. Jaundice and clinical features resembling cholestasis are commonly present. The prognosis is generally good and fulminant hepatitis is rarely seen with mixed injury. The main drugs associated with mixed injury include tricyclic antidepressants, NSAIDs, macrolides, nitrofurantoin, sulindac, sulfonamides, amoxicillin/clavulanate, cyclosporine, methimazole and carbamazepine.

Table 6.8: Drugs causing mixed liver injury

Amitriptyline
Amoxicillin clavulanic acid
Ampicillin
Captopril
Carbamazepine
Cimetidine
Cotrimoxazole
Flutamide
Ibuprofen
Naproxen
Nitrofurantoin
Phenylbutazone
Quinidine
Ranitidine
Sulfonamides
Sulindac

Chronic hepatitis: Drug induced chronic hepatitis affects more females than males and is usually accompanied by serologic autoimmune markers. Drugs associated with drug induced chronic hepatitis include dantrolene, diclofenac, methyldopa, minocycline, nitrofurantoin and sulfonamides. Drug induced liver damage occurs after drug administration for a prolonged period and beyond the initial liver insult. In patients with chronic hepatitis due to drug therapy accompanied by serologic markers of autoimmune disease, the majority of these patients (>90%) are women. In contrast, drugs such as lisinopril and trazodone are implicated in drug induced chronic hepatitis without the serologic markers of autoimmune disease. Agents such as acetaminophen, aspirin and dantrolene produce chronic hepatitis through toxic effects of the drugs, rather than through chronic inflammation of the hepatocytes. Clinical presentation of drug induced chronic hepatitis has characteristics of both acute and chronic hepatic injury, such as enlarged liver, splenomegaly and ascites. Jaundice, anorexia, and fatigue are also common. Results of liver function tests are usually elevated and coagulopathy is often present. Withdrawal of the responsible agent may lead to improvement and complete resolution of chronic hepatitis within weeks. However, continued therapy with these agents may lead to cirrhosis, fulminant hepatic failure and death.

Chronic steatosis: In contrast to acute steatosis associated with therapeutic agents, chronic steatosis has a minimal number of clinical manifestations. A macrovesicular pattern, in which a single large vacuole of fat fills the hepatocyte and displaces the nucleus to the periphery, is seen in this form of steatosis. Enlargement of the liver is the primary clinical feature of this form of chronic fatty degeneration and often results from the prolonged use of drugs such as glucocorticoids, methotrexate, amiodarone and tamoxifen. Most of the cases of chronic steatosis is benign, whereas methotrexate induced steatosis can progress to cirrhosis. In addition, valproic acid has been associated with fatty degeneration that can result in chronic liver failure and severe hepatic necrosis.

Other forms of drug induced liver injury: (Table 6.9-6.13) Other types of drug induced reactions that result in liver injury include granulomatous hepatitis, vascular injury and hepatic tumor. Clinical characteristics of granulomatous reactions include fever, malaise, headache and myalgia manifesting 10 days to four months after the initiation of drug therapy, with splenomegaly presenting in up to 15% of cases. Up to 60 medications have been associated with hepatic granulomas. In the vascular injury type of hepatotoxicity, hepatic vein thrombosis and hepatic venous occlusion can occur from drug therapy. Clinical symptoms of hepatic vein thrombosis include hepatomegaly, abdominal pain, ascites and jaundice. Although rare, this type of liver injury has been associated with oral contraceptives. Hepatic venous occlusion also causes similar clinical presentation and has been associated with chemotherapeutic agents such as etoposide, vincristine, vinblastine, azathioprine, cyclophosphamide, methotrexate and mitomycin. Drug induced liver tumors rarely occur but are clearly associated with oral contraceptives and anabolic steroids. Incidence of oral contraceptive–induced hepatic tumors is estimated to be between three and four cases per 100,000 exposed women annually.

Table 6.9: Drugs associated with hepatic granulomas

Allopurinol Nitrofurantoin
Para-amino Salicylic and Oral Contraceptive Pills
Carbamazepine Penicillin
Cephalexin Phenylbutazone
Clofibrate Phenytoin
Diazepam Procainamide
Diltiazem Procarbazine
Erythromycin Estolate Quinidine
Gold Salt Silicone
Halothane Starch
Hydralazine Sulfasalazine
INH Sulfonamide
Methyldopa Sulfonylurea Derivatives
Metolazone Talc

Table 6.10: Drugs causing veno-occlusive disease

Azathioprine
Carmustine
Doxorubicin
6-mercaptopurine
6-thioguanine
Vincristine

Table 6.11: Drugs associated with Budd-Chiari syndrome

Arsenical derivatives
Cyclophosphamide
Dacarbazine
Oral contraceptive pills
Vincristine

Table 6.12: Drugs associated with peliosis hepatitis

Anabolic steroid
Androgens
Arsenical derivatives
Corticosteroids
Medroxy progesterone
Tamoxifen
6-Thioguanine

Table 6.13: Drugs associated with neoplasm

Anabolic steroid
Androgens
Oral contraceptive pills
Anabolic steroids
Methotrexate
Oral contraceptive pills
Oral Hypoglycemic agents
Thorium – dioxide
Anabolic steroids
Androgens
Arsenical derivatives
Oral contraceptive pills
Cholagiocarcinoma
Anabolic steroids
Androgens
Methyldopa
Oral contraceptive pills

SPECIFIC DRUG RELATED HEPATITIS

Antitubercular Drugs

The hepatotoxicity of individual antitubercular drugs is not well studied, since these drugs are invariably used in combination. Streptomycin and ethambutol are not hepatotoxic, but isoniazid, rifampicin, pyrazinamide and PAS can cause liver injury.

Isoniazid

Two distinct types of hepatic reactions are identified with isoniazid. In more than 10% of all patients who take isoniazid a mild, subclinical, non-specific focal hepatitis occurs within the first few weeks to months of drug administration. It is manifested by an increase in serum aminotransferases which most often return to normal even if the drug is continued. Though less common in children, the injury occurs in all age groups and has no clear relationship to sex, ethnic background or the rate at which isoniazid is acetylated in the liver.

In about 1% of individuals, an overt hepatitis like illness develops. The time of onset of hepatitis is quite variable, about 50% of cases occur within 2 months whereas in a few onset may be delayed to 12 months. Patients in whom onset is delayed or in whom the drug is continued after hepatitis has set in, are the most severely affected. It may present with flu like syndrome, progressive jaundice or severe acute liver failure. The treatment includes immediate stoppage of the drug. Prevention or early detection remains elusive. Routine monitoring of aminotransferases is of little help as there is no defined level which would detect the early lesion reliably. Patient should report if symptoms of intercurrent illness appear.

The mechanism of hepatotoxicity is by the formation of toxic reactive intermediates. Earlier studies suggesting that rapid acetylators of isoniazid are at a greater risk of develop hepatic injury have not been confirmed.

Rifampicin

Rifampicin is used in combination with isoniazid. Hepatic injury occurring in the first month of combination therapy is attributed to rifampicin in contrast to isoniazid injury which occurs late. The exact incidence is uncertain due to combination with other drugs. A high incidence was noted in smaller studies but in contrast, in 379 patients treated daily with isoniazid 300 mg and rifampicin 600 mg did not observe any hepatitis. The incidence is higher in children with tubercular meningitis or in malnourished children. It has been suggested that rifampicin induces microsomal drug metabolism, it may predispose to a severe and rapidly appearing form of isoniazid induced hepatitis.

Once patient develops hepatitis, drugs should be withdrawn. Patients should be put on streptomycin and ethambutol till aminotransferases normalize. There is a little information available on how to reintroduce isoniazid and rifampicin. Generally isoniazid could be started in lower doses of 5 mg/kg/day and rifampicin is added a week later after the introduction of isoniazid, if enzymes remain normal.

Pyrazinamide

There is now adequate experience with modern short course regimens containing pyrazinamide. There is no report of a high incidence of hepatotoxicity with pyrazinamide regimens.

Psychotropic Drugs

Chlorpromazine(CPZ) and other neuroleptics, including haloperidol tend to produce cholestatic lesions. Jaundice occurs in 5-10% of all patients who receive chlorpromazine. Re-administration of small doses leads to prompt recurrence of hepatic dysfunction or jaundice in approximately half the patients. Prodromal symptoms which occur in 75% of patients and may include lever, chills, abdominal pain. Eosinophilia occurs in about 60% of cases. The hepatic injury is mainly cholestatic or mixed, rarely hepatocellular. Severe itching is common. Serum alkaline phosphatase is raised and aminotransferases mildly elevated. Prognosis is good as two thirds recover within 8 weeks and the remainder in 12 months.

Among the monoamine oxidase inhibiting derivatives of hydrazine, iproniazid is the most widely recognized as a hepatotoxic drug. It produces acute viral hepatitis like injury. Benzodiazepines, the commonly used tranquilizers, appear to have a very low hepatotoxic potential. Chlordiazepoxide, diazepam and flurazepam have been associated with cholestasis in a few cases only. There is no hepatotoxicity with midazolam.

Anticonvulsants

Chronic phenytoin use is associated with altered liver function tests, acute hepatitis (4-6 weeks after start of therapy) or hepatic encephalopathy. Treatment is supportive corticosteroids may improve the systemic and serum sickness like symptoms, but not the course of the disease.

Valproic acid is well tolerated but leads to asymptomatic liver enzyme elevation in 11-12% cases after 10-12 weeks of therapy. Clinically overt hepatitis is less common. Carbamazepine also causes hepatic injury, mostly a glaucomatous reaction.

Antimicrobials

Erythromycin estolate (also ethylsuccinate and lactobionate) is commonly associated with cholestatic reaction and significant portal inflammation and focal hepatic necrosis. Occurs more often in adults. Sulfonamides, tetracycline and nitrofurantoin are also associated with different types of hepatotoxicity.

Hormones and Allied Drugs

Oral contraceptives cause cholestatic injury, pruritis and jaundice within first two months of treatment. Fever, rash and arthralgia is absent. Prothrombin time is normal. After stoppage of the drug the syndrome rapidly resolves. Oral contraceptives may be associated with hepatic adenoma, focal nodular hyperplasia and hepatocellular carcinoma.

Analgesics and Anti-inflammatory Drugs

Acetaminophen

After moderate to massive (>15 g) quantities of ingestion of acetaminophen, acute hepatic injury may develop. Initially there is a "latent period" of about 24 hours during which nausea, vomiting and diaphoresis occurs. This is followed by acute hepatocellular necrosis characterized by tender hepatomegaly, jaundice and liver encephalopathy. The toxic intermediate metabolite is N-acetyle-p-benzoquinone imine (NAPQI).

The threshold dose of hepatotoxicity varies inversely with the hepatic glutathione stores. Fasting and ethanol decrease glutathione. N-acetyl-cysteine is the drug of choice and gives best result if given within first 10 hours of injury.

Aspirin

Aspirin induced liver injury is most commonly seen in chronic rheumatoid arthritis treated for several weeks with high dose of aspirin. They manifest with raised enzymes and less commonly with subclinical hyper-bilirubinemia. Aspirin may predispose to development of Reye's syndrome when given in a viral infection in children.

Methotrexate

Chronic methotrexate therapy given in psoriasis leads to hepatic fibrosis. The incidence of cirrhosis is low with a total cumulative dose below 1.5 g.

6-Mercaptopurine and Azathioprine

Both agents cause dose dependent hepatotoxicity, mainly cholestatic, rarely hepatocellular. The lesion is reversible on stopping the drug.

Halothane

Halothane is metabolized in two different ways by oxidation and reduction via cytochrome P_{450}. Reductive metabolism in the presence of low oxygen leads to free radical production and lipid peroxidation. Oxidation forms trifluoroacetythalide. These proteins appear on the surface of hepatocytes against which antibodies develop. The clinical toxicity appears to be immune mediated.

Incidence of halothane hepatitis increases among patient undergoing repeated anesthesia. Symptoms appear several days to two to three weeks after exposure. This interval is reduces to few days when there is previous exposure to halothane. Clinical picture may vary from fever, jaundice, tender hepatomegaly to signs of liver failure including ascites.

Risk Factors

Numerous factors such as age, sex, genetic predisposition and degree of alcohol consumption appear to increase the susceptibility of DILD to variety of therapeutic agents. Although patients with mild to moderate chronic liver disease do not appear to be at increased risk of hepatic injury from therapeutic compounds, certain drugs, including methotrexate, tolcapone, niacin and pemoline, should be used with caution in these patients, since they may have altered metabolism of these agents and may be at increased risk for liver injury.

Most hepatic adverse effects associated with drugs occur in adults rather than children. In the adult population, persons more than 40 years are at increased risk for DILD. This may be due to increased frequency of drug exposure, multiple drug therapy and age related changes in drug metabolism. Reports indicate that drug-induced liver injury occurs at a higher rate in patients older than 50 years and that drug associated jaundice occurs in up to 20% of the geriatric population. In general, female gender has been associated with an increased risk of hepatic dysfunction due to drugs, especially from agents such as nitrofurantoin, methyldopa and sulfonamides.

A familial predisposition to drug-induced hepatic injury is rare but has been reported with drugs such as phenytoin. Genetic factors in affected individuals may decrease the ability to metabolize or eliminate drugs or may decrease the ability to modulate the immune response to drugs or metabolites. Chronic, excessive ingestion of alcohol may also increase the risk of hepatotoxicity from drugs such as acetaminophen by lowering the glutathione store and inhibiting clearance of toxic metabolites. Alcohol may also predispose many drugs to hepatotoxicity. Such agents include acetaminophen, isoniazid, methotrexate and vitamin A.

Herbal Medication Induced Liver Injury

As herbal remedies continue to gain popularity, an increasing number of hepatic injuries due to herbal drugs are being reported. Liver injuries from herbal remedies range from mild and self-limiting to life-threatening conditions such as liver failure. The spectrum of herbal remedy induced liver disease encompasses all forms of hepatic injuries, including minor elevation in liver function test results, acute and chronic hepatitis, steatosis, cholestasis, hepatic necrosis, hepatic fibrosis, veno-occlusive disease and acute liver failure. While these agents are readily available, they are not subjected to rigorous testing or regulation and a standardized manufacturing process does not exist. Consequently, safety information on these products is not available to the public. Potential health risks are increased with widespread use of these agents.

Comfrey is often ingested as an ingredient in herbal teas and belongs to species of plants that produce pyrrolizidine alkaloids, which have been recognized for more than 70 years as a cause of hepatotoxicity. The principal form of liver injury with comfrey is veno-occlusive disease, characterized by nonthrombotic occlusion of small veins within the liver lobules. Liver failure has occurred during the acute phase, with a mortality rate of up to 40%.

Jin bu huan is a traditional herbal remedy that has been used as a sedative and an analgesic. At least 10 cases of acute hepatitis have been linked to the use of Jin bu huan, with patients presenting with symptoms of fever, fatigue, nausea, pruritis, abdominal pain, jaundice and hepatomegaly. Symptoms resolve after the withdrawal of the agent in most cases. Kava has been one of the most popular herbal remedies in recent years and is usually used for anxiety, insomnia and stress. Several cases of kava-associated hepatotoxicity, including one report of hepatic failure requiring liver transplantation have been reported. Warnings of potential health risks associated with the use of kava have been issued by the FDA. Other herbal remedies implicated in hepatic injury include chaparral leaf, camphor, gentian, germander and valerian.

Diagnosis of Drug Induced Liver Injury

It is an exclusive diagnose–excluded other causes:

- Relate drugs to onset of illness.
- Look for preexisting liver disease.
- Clinical examination, previous laboratory investigations.
- Consider alternate causes:
  - Viral Hepatitis—Serological markers.
  - Biliary disease—Ultrasound examination.
  - Observe the effects of stopping drugs.
  - Liver biopsy—Suspected pre-exiting liver disease.
  - Challenge test with drugs—Never.

Treatment and Prevention

The only well established treatment method to prevent drug-induced hepatitis is administering N-acetylcysteine to detoxify reactive metabolites, which can be given to patients with acetaminophen overdose. N-acetylcysteine should be given within the first 10 hours for the optimal protective effect. In other cases of drug associated hepatic injury, there is no specific treatment. Identifying and stopping the administration of the offending agent is the most important step in preventing the injury from progressing to life-threatening condition.

Prevention of drug-induced liver injury begins with assessing the toxicity of the drug at the preclinical stage and analyzing the safety in healthy volunteers or in patients during the various steps of drug development. While these measures are currently used in drug development, hepatotoxicity continues to occur although at low frequency in susceptible patients.

After the drug is marketed, prevention of hepatic injury can be accomplished by avoiding readministration of the offending drug and other drugs belonging to the same class. There are several reported cases of cross-hepatotoxicity between drugs within the same class, such as NSAIDs, macrolides, sulfonamides, tricyclic antidepressants and phenothiazine derivatives. In addition, avoiding the simultaneous administration of several drugs can also prevent drug induced liver injury. Drugs associated with enzyme induction or inhibition can produce drug–drug interactions when administered with substrates of these reactions, which can result in hepatic injury. The elderly require a higher level of monitoring since older individuals are more susceptible to drug hepatotoxicity. Codeine sulphate and loperamide may be avoided as it may precipitate hepatic encephalopathy. Spironolactone is a safer diuretic in liver diseases. Paracetamol is relatively safer than aspirin.

Finally, follow-up liver function tests should be routinely monitored, especially for drugs with a known association to liver injury. But, liver function tests may have limited valve with some drugs. Transient rise of transaminases are common in 5-20% of cases. Drugs like methotrexate and amiodarone can produce extensive liver damage before raising the enzymes.

Drug related liver injuries are increasingly becoming important to specialists in all spheres of medicine. This assumes greater significance in developing countries like India where a poor nutritional status and a high rate of infections like tuberculosis may increase the chances of drug related liver injuries. It is also necessary to study the genetic polymorphism of commonly used drugs in different populations. Since there are only a few specific therapies for drug hepatitis, a high index of suspicion and early withdrawal of the offering agent should remain the hallmark of management of these patients.

CHAPTER SEVEN

Renal ADRs

Drugs may cause a variety of renal disorders including acute renal failure, chronic renal failure and the nephrotic syndrome. Recognition of drugs as a cause of renal disease is of particular importance because such lesions are reversible if the drug is stopped. It has been estimated that 5-10 % of all renal diseases are due to drug therapy.

The addition of newer drugs, besides contributing to better therapeutic potential, has added another dimension to the causation of renal disease the abuse or indiscriminate use of drugs, coupled with easy availability has taken its toll on the kidneys. The kidney falls prey to the drug's onslaught because of properties of kidney which make it susceptible to injury.

The kidneys are prone to drug induced injury for a variety of reasons. The main reasons are:
a. High blood flow.
b. The presence of active metabolic products.
c. Medullary concentration of some substances.

A list of important drugs causing renal injury is shown in Table 7.1.

The kidney is an organ characterized by a large volume of blood supply (20-25% of the cardiac output) which ensures a high level of toxicant delivery over a period of time. The extensive reabsorptive capacity of the tubule with specialised transporters promotes cellular uptake of the toxicant. Concentrating capability of the tubule produces high concentrations in the medullary lumen and interstitium. High metabolic rates and workload increases the sensitivity to toxicants. Metabolic alteration (biotransformation enzymes) may produce highly toxic metabolites or reactive intermediates.

The nephrotoxic chemicals damage specific portions of tubule with the brunt being borne by the proximal tubule. Segment specific targets exist for nephrotoxicants. The reasons for segmental specific nephrotoxicity of agents may be attributable to the differences in toxicant delivery, differences in transport and uptake among segments and differences in biotransformation among segments. The end result of the nephrotoxicants effect on the epithelial cell is cell injury and death. Cell death could be the consequence of ischemia related to a decreased renal blood flow. Intraluminal tubular obstruction (increases the Intraluminal pressure and decreases single nephron glomerular filtration rate), "backleak" of tubular infiltrate (due to loss of epithelial cells) and inhibition of cellular repair and regeneration are processes, other than cell death, that could contribute to drug related acute renal dysfunction.

Table 7.1: Established causes of drug induced nephrotoxicity

Acute Renal Failure	
1. Pre-renal	Non-steroidal anti inflammatory drugs
2. Intrinsic a. Toxic tubular cell Injury b. Interstitial nephritis	 Aminoglycosides, cephalosporin iodinated radiological contrast materials Cyclosporine A Methoxyflurane Methicillin, rifampicin, furosemide sulfonamides
Obstructive renal failure	Sulfonamides, methysergide
Chronic renal failure (Due to chronic interstitial Nephritis or chronic Glomerulonephritis)	Analgesics Heroin Amphetamines
Nephrotic Syndrome	Gold Penicillamine Captopril Non steroidal anti-inflammatory drugs

Drugs were reported to cause 18.3% of acute renal failure in a one year survey. In India a study reported a 20% incidence of drug induced acute renal failure with a large proportion (40%) secondary to aminoglycosides usage. Two aspects of the relationship between drugs and the kidney are of clinical importance:

1. Some drugs are nephrotoxic.
2. While pharmacokinetics of other drugs may be altered by renal diseases.

While these two problems maybe related in clinical practice, they are best discussed separately.

A. NEPHROTOXIC DRUGS CAUSING VARIOUS RENAL ABNORMALITIES

1. ACUTE RENAL FAILURE

Pre-renal ARF

Non steroidal anti-inflammatory drugs (NSAIDs) act by inhibiting the enzyme cyclooxygenase, which catalyzes the formation of prostaglandins from arachidonic acid. When intra renal levels of the vasoconstrictor angiotensin are high, as in volume depletion, cardiac failure, cirrhosis, nephrotic syndrome and renal failure, there is often a compensatory increase in the renal synthesis of vasodilator prostaglandins. Acute inhibition by NSAIDs therefore will lead to reduced renal blood flow with consequent reduction in the glomerular filtration rate in susceptible individuals. Renal impairment is reversible within 8-48 hrs if treatment with the offending drug is discontinued.

There are two mechanisms by which drugs may cause intrinsic ARF:

a. Toxic Renal Tubular Injury and
b. Acute Interstitial Nephritis.

A. Toxic Tubular Injury

Toxic tubular injury is caused by many agents like aminoglycosides antibiotics, first generation cephalosporins, amphotericin-B, cisplatin and cyclosporine-A.

Aminoglycosides

Aminoglycosides cause damage by binding to acidic phospholipids in the proximal tubules of the renal cortex. This group of drugs is probably the most common cause of drug related ARF. Gentamicin is more toxic than tobramycin and neomycin. Acute renal failure due to aminoglycosides is non-oliguric and occurs 7-10 days after the initiation of treatment. Elderly patients and those with pre-existing renal disease are more prone to amino glycoside nephrotoxicity. Concomitant administration of drugs like furosemide and cephalosporin increases the incidence of nephrotoxicity. Renal failure is reversible if identified early and the offending agent is withdrawn. As the renal failure is non-oliguric it is necessary to monitor blood urea and serum creatinine levels regularly.

Cephalosporin

Toxic tubular damage is associated with the use of the first generation compounds like cephaloridine and cephalothin. However, this is not a problem with the newer cephalosporin like cefotaxime and cefuroxime.

Tetracyclines

Proximal tubular damage was a common side effect of the older tetracyclines but does not occur with the newer tetracyclines. Nephrogenic diabetes insipidus is a specific effect of demeclocycline use. In patients with renal impairment, tetracyclines cause blood urea to rise by their antianabolic effect. Doxycycline is safe in renal failure.

Amphotericin B

The nephrotoxic effects of amphotericin-B are acute renal failure, distal renal tubular acidosis, wasting of potassium by the renal tubules and nephrogenic diabetes insipidus. Toxicity is dose dependent. Renal impairment is usually not reversible and defects in distal tubular function may persist for long periods.

B. Acute Interstitial Nephritis

Many drugs may cause an acute deterioration in renal function due to an inflammatory process in the interstitium. The mechanism is usually thought to be immediate hypersensitivity. Clinically this manifests as fever, skin rash and eosinophilia. Red blood cells and eosinophils appear in the urine and may be detected by staining of the urinary sediment with Wright's stain. However, renal failure may be the only feature and it is important therefore, to consider drug induced acute interstitial nephritis as a possibility in any patient with acute renal failure. The agents which most commonly cause acute interstitial nephritis are penicillin, rifampicin, furosemide, NSAIDs, allopurinol and cimetidine. Histological, there is marked interstitial oedema and a patchy or diffuse inflammatory cell infiltrate usually composed of mononuclear cells. The glomeruli are relatively unaffected.

Once the diagnosis is established, discontinuation of the offending agent is mandatory. The role of steroids is controversial. Most patients recover adequate renal function whether or not steroids are given, but there is some evidence that return of renal function is quicker as well as more complete in those receiving steroids.

2. OBSTRUCTIVE ACUTE RENAL FAILURE

Obstruction of the distal tubules and collecting ducts by precipitates of uric acid has been described in patients with hematological malignancies treated with cytotoxic drugs. Treatment is preventive. Patients with large tumour loads should be pretreated with allopurinol. Adequate hydration should be maintained and urine alkalinized during administration of cytotoxic therapy. Methysergide occasionally used in the treatment of migraine causes retroperitoneal fibrosis which may produce ureteric obstruction.

3. CHRONIC RENAL FAILURE

The two major mechanisms by which drugs cause chronic renal failure are chronic interstitial nephritis and chronic glomerulonephritis.

Chronic Interstitial Nephritis

Analgesic Nephropathy

This disease is caused by chronic ingestion of combinations of analgesic preparations usually containing phenacetin and aspirin. Aspirin, phenacetin or paracetamol when given alone are unlikely to cause clinically significant nephropathy. Pathologically the earliest change is patchy necrosis of cells in the papillae followed by an inflammatory cell infiltrate and papillary necrosis. The pathogenesis is obscure, but may be due to toxic metabolites of phenacetin

Toxic damage to papillary structure leads to papillary necrosis and inflammatory changes in the rest of the kidney. The incidence of this condition varies greatly in various countries, reflecting differences in analgesic consumption and availability. Diagnosis is made on the basis of a clinical history of analgesic abuse, profound anemia, characteristic radiological abnormalities, the presence of papillary tissue in the urine and renal histology.

Lithium therapy may cause chronic interstitial nephritis, although this is a rare event.

Chronic Glomerulonephritis:

Heroin addicts may develop a form of glomerulonephritis histologically resembling focal glomerular sclerosis or membranoproliferative glomerulonephritis. The prognosis for continued renal function is poor and the pathogenesis unknown. Amphetamine abuse may result in a condition resembling polyarteritis nodosa.

4. NEPHROTIC SYNDROME

A variety of drugs can produce the nephrotic syndrome e.g. gold, penicillamine and captopril being the best known causative agents. Nephrotic syndrome occurs in 1-3 percent of rheumatoid patients treated with gold salts. The histological pattern is usually that of membranous glomerulonephritis. Renal function is usually normal and the lesion regresses after cessation of therapy, although it may take several months to do so. Gold therapy should be discontinued in rheumatoid patients who develop proteinuria. Penicillamine and captopril may also cause membranous nephropathy.

B. DRUGS CAUSING RENAL DISEASE DUE TO ALTERED PHARMACOKINETICS

Patients with renal failure may often have to be treated with drugs that are intended to be used in patients with normal renal function. Obviously, drugs excreted mainly through the kidney will produce greater plasma concentrations and will maintains these levels for longer periods in patients with renal failure than in patients with normal renal function. Also, certain patients with renal failure often react atypically and unpredictably to a number of pharmacologic agents. Therefore the side effects of a drug may be related to factors other than drug concentration. Alert, attentive and careful monitoring of drug therapy is absolutely necessary in patients with renal failure.

Pharmacokinetics in Patients with Renal Failure

Patients with renal failure, display altered pharmacokinetics due to the following reasons:
1. Decreased absorption.
2. Alteration in plasma protein binding.
3. Impairment of drug metabolism.
4. Decreased renal clearance.

Modification of Drug Dosage in Renal Failure

In therapeutics, it is important to determine the range, in terms of plasma concentration of the drug, between the effective dose of a drug and the dose that induces toxic reactions.

In adjusting the dosage for patients with renal failure the initial loading dose usually needs little or no reduction.

A few notable exceptions to this principle are digoxin and morphine (because of changes in distribution volume and sensitivity). After the initial dose achieves the peak plasma concentration, the plasma level will decrease more slowly i.e. the half life will be prolonged in proportion to the severity of renal failure as reflected by the plasma creatinine concentration. The prolonged half life means that the plasma concentration will be higher than usual when the next dose is due.

A marked reduction in dosage will be required when the kidney is the only route of excretion of a drug and renal failure is severe. Obviously the half lives of those drugs eliminated predominantly by extrarenal routes will be affected little by renal failure and intermediate effects will result when elimination is partially renal. The fractional elimination by the kidney (the renal clearance as a fraction of total plasma clearance) determines the extent of dosage adjustment required in renal failure.

Table 7.2: Dose reduction in renal insufficiency

Drug	Dosage (mg/kg)	
	Normal	Severe renal failure
1. Penicillin	5- 100/8 hrly	1-5/12 hrly
2. Ampicillin	7/6 hrly	4/6 hrly
3. Amoxicillin	10/8 hrly	7/12 hrly
4. Cloxacillin	7/6 hrly	7/8 hrly
5. Carbenicillin	50/4 hrly	30/12 hrly

Calculation of Dose

Elimination of a drug is linearly related to GFR which is best expressed clinically as the creatinine clearance that can be obtained from the following formula (Cockroft Gault equation):

$$\text{Male: CLcr} = \frac{140 - \text{Age}}{\text{Ccr}} \times \frac{\text{Weight}}{72}\ \text{ml/min}$$

$$\text{Female: CLcr} = 0.85\,\frac{140 - \text{Age}}{\text{Ccr}} \times \frac{\text{Weight}}{72}\ \text{ml/min}$$

(Ccr=serum creatinine)

Dose can be calculated as:

$$\text{Dose in renal insufficiency} = \text{Doses} \times \frac{\text{CLcr}}{100}$$

This is the basis upon which drugs are categorized as requiring little or no dosage modification, modest adjustment or marked reduction in renal failure.

Dose Reduction with Specific Drugs (Table 7.2)

Chemotherapeutic Drugs

Nephrotoxicity has become a major complication of antibiotic therapy particularly in patients with renal failure. Many antibiotics have a narrow margin of safety and since most are excreted by the kidney their accumulation in renal failure can induce or increase toxicity.

All agents of the aminoglycoside group are nephrotoxic and ototoxic. The loading dose is the same in patients with or without renal failure subsequently therapeutic levels are maintained by a combination of dosage or interval adjustment methods e.g. gentamicin is given to patients without renal failure in doses of 1.0-1.5 mg/kg once every 5-8 hours and to patients with severe renal failure in doses of 0.5-1.0 mg/kg every 72 hours.

Cephalosporin may be nephrotoxic in combination with aminoglycosides antibiotics or diuretics and when the patient is dehydrated. An example of the dosage schedules: Cephalexin, normally given in doses of 15 mg/kg every 6 hours is given in doses of 7 mg/kg every 24 hours to patients with severe renal failure.

With penicillins, allergic interstitial nephritis may occur. Seizures and coagulopathy can occur at high blood levels. For those with renal failure, half the usual dose of chloroquine should be given. No supplemental doses are required after haemodialysis.

Chloramphenicol is eliminated mostly by hepatic

metabolism. In renal failure full doses can be utilised but the bone marrow in uraemic patients is more susceptible to inhibition. With erythromycin dosage adjustment is not required. With metronidazole, gastrointestinal symptoms may mimic uremia. The dosage interval has to be increased to 12-24 hours in those with severe renal failure. Supplemental doses are required after haemodialysis. Methamine mandelate, nalidixic acid and nitrofurantoin are best avoided in patients with renal failure. Trimethoprim may increase serum creatinine by competition for renal secretion. It achieves adequate urine levels even in those patients with low GFR. In those with severe renal failure the dose needs to be given only once in 24 hours.

Amphotericin B is nephrotoxic and in severe renal failure the dosage interval needs to be prolonged to 36 hours. No supplemental dosage is required after dialysis. Because of long term use, excessive accumulation of antituberculous drugs may induce toxicity.

Sedatives and Hypnotics

These drugs are eliminated by the liver and when used in renal failure do not require any dosage adjustment or supplementation after dialysis (unexceptional in pentazocin which requires supplement after haemodialysis).

These agents however, may cause excessive sedation and respiratory depression in uraemic patients. All barbiturates may cause excessive sedation and may increase osteomalacia in patients with end stage renal disease (ESRD). Phenobarbital and thiopental require dose adjustment in renal failure and supplementation after haemodialysis. The dosage interval of phenobarbital needs to be increased to 12-16 hours and the thiopental dose should be reduced to 75% in those with severe renal failure. Benzodiazepines may cause excessive sedation and encephalopathy in ESRD patients. Chlordiazepoxide and diazepam need no dosage adjustment. Lorazepam doses need to be reduced to half the usual and oxazepam to 75% in patients with severe renal failure. Haloperidol, chlorpromazine, amitriptyline, doxepine, imipramine and nortryptyline do not need dose adjustments or post dialysis supplementation when used to treat those with renal failure.

Anticonvulsants

Phenytoin and sodium valproate do not need dose adjustment or postdialysis supplementation. A carbamazepine dose should be reduced to 75% of the usual dose.

Analgesics and Anti-inflammatory Drugs

With acetaminophen and paracetamol the dosage interval should be increased to 8 hours in patients with severe renal failure. Aspirin may decrease GFR in conditions such as CHF, SLE etc. Renal blood flow is prostaglandin dependent and may add to uraemic gastrointestinal and hematological symptoms. It is prudent to avoid its use in those with severe renal failure. Ibuprofen, fenoprofen, naproxen, indomethacin and piroxicam when used in renal failure do not require any dosage adjustment.

Hypoglycemic Agents

Chlorpropamide produces prolonged hypoglycemia in azotemic patients and should be avoided in patients with renal failure. Glibenclamide, glipizide and tolbutamide need no dosage adjustment. Insulin has a prolonged half-life in patients with renal failure and dosage reduction to half of the usual dose is indicated when renal failure develops.

GIT Drugs

H_2 blockers (Cimetidine, ranitidine and fomatidine) increase serum creatinine and decrease creatinine clearance by inhibition of renal tubular secretion. They may cause mental confusion in patients with renal failure. Acute renal failure is reported with their use. The dose should be reduced to half of the usual dose, and the dosage interval should be increased to 12 hours. Metoclopramide requires a dose reduction to half of the usual dose in patients with severe renal disease.

CVS Drugs

With antihypertensive drugs the blood pressure reading is the best guide to dose and interval adjustment. When antiarrhythmics drugs are used blood levels help to guide therapy in ESRD. Lidocaine dosage requires no alterations in renal failure. In severe renal failure the dosage intervals of procainamide should be increased to 8-24 hours. In severe renal disease plasma levels of quinidine increase, so doses need to be reduced. In the case of disopyramide the dose interval should be increased to 24-40 hours in severe renal failures. Cardiac glycosides add to uraemic gastrointestinal symptoms. Serum levels are the best guide to dosage and should be measured about 10 hours after drug administration. Digitoxin is mainly eliminated by the hepatic route, hence no dosage adjustment is needed. The loading dose in the case of digoxin should be decreased by 50% in ESRD. The maintenance dose should be reduced to 10-25% of usual dose or the interval increased to 48 hours in severe renal failure. Calcium channel blocking drugs may cause headache, flushing and dizziness especially in renal failure. Nifedipine may cause oedema. No alteration in dosage is required with renal failure.

All Diuretics produce extracellular volume depletion. Acetazolamide may potentiate acidosis and can induce calcium urothiasis and hypokalemia. It is ineffective in severe renal failure and should not be used. Thiazides are not useful in severe renal failure and have undesirable side effects like hypokalemia, hyperuricemia and metabolic alkalosis. It is prudent to avoid their use in the presence of renal failure. Loop of Henle blocking drugs are ototoxic and potentiate aminoglycosides nephrotoxicity. Bumetanide produces gynecomastia and muscle weakness. It requires no dosage alteration.

Ethacrynic acid produces severe deafness in renal failure and should be avoided. Furosemide may be helpful in high doses in the presence of end stage renal failure. Potassium sparing diuretics may produce hypokalemia especially in diabetics. In addition amiloride can produce hyperchloremic metabolic acidosis. Spironolactone may produce gynecomastia and impotence and triametrene can cause folate antagonism and renal calculi formation. This group of diuretics should be avoided in the presence of renal failure.

Table 7.3: Drug induced toxic renal syndromes

Acute Renal Failure	*Examples*
• Prerenal (decreased perfusion)	Diuretics, NSAIDs, ACE Inhibitor
• Intrinsic Renal (direct tubule cell toxicity)	Aminoglycosides, Radiocontrast Media, Cisplatin
Acute tubular necrosis	
• Hemolysis	Quinine, sulfonamides, hydralazine
• Rhabdomyolysis	Lovastatin, ethanol, barbiturate
• Acute Interstitial Nephritis (Immune-mediated)	Penicillin, rifampicin, sulfonamides
TTP-HUS	
(Vascular endothelial injury)	Cyclosporine, tacrolimus, quinine
• Obstructive	Acyclovir, methotrexate, sulfonamides
• Intratubular	Methysergide, methyldopa, gold
• Ureteral (retroperitoneal fibrosis)	Penicillamine, captopril, NSAIDs mercury
Nephrotic Syndrome (immune-mediated) ***Renal Tubular** Dysfunction* ***Chronic Renal Failure*** (Interstitial failure) NSAIDs, Acetaminophen	

Nephrotoxicity of Specific Drugs and Prevention

NSAIDs

The number of patients at risk or affected by the nephrotoxic properties of NSAIDs has increased with the widespread usage of this class of drugs. The mechanisms of nephrotoxicity relate to the capacity to induce vasomotor changes and a reduction in renal function. Additionally nephrotic syndrome associated with interstitial nephritis, chronic renal injury and water electrolyte abnormalities (sodium, potassium and water) are encountered. The common thread through all these syndromes seems to be a disruption of prostaglandin metabolism.

The occurrence of the nephrotoxic syndromes are related to the presence of risk factors in the subset of patients, the patient with a decreased effective arterial blood volume (congestive heart failure, cirrhosis, nephrotic syndrome, sepsis, haemorrhage, diuretic therapy, 'third-spacing", volume depletion/hypotension) as well as those with normal, or increased effective arterial volume (chronic renal failure, glomerulonephritis, elderly, contrast-induced nephropathy and cyclosporine) are at risk of developing vasomotor renal failure. The association of a nephrotic state with interstitial nephritis characterizes the toxicity of NSAIDs. Analgesic nephropathy has been found to be a consequence of chronic NSAIDs intake. Combination of drugs may potentiate the nephrotoxic properties and enhance the risk of toxicity. Aspirin and NSAIDs combination produce an increased risk of renal failure and hence are not encouraged.

Table 7.4: Preventing NSAID nephrotoxicity

1. Recognize the potential (situational factor) for causation of nephrotoxicity and take corrective action to minimize nephrotoxic potential.
2. Avoid chronic (habitual) use of NSAIDs.
3. Avoid combinations of analgesics.
4. Monitoring use of drugs when consumption is mandatory. Low dose aspirin safe (as used for prevention of cardio-vascular events).
5. All available analgesics have a nephrotoxic potential (except paracetamol) and should be carefully considered before usage.

Antibiotics

Antibiotic associated renal failure is predominantly noted with the use of aminoglycosides antibiotics though it may also occur with beta Lactam, vancomycin, sulfonamides and antifungal antibiotics. A few factors may also predispose to nephrotoxicity viz., repeated courses of aminoglycosides a few months apart, malnutrition and high trough concentrations.

Table 7.5: Modifiable and non-modifiable risk factors for aminoglycosides nephrotoxicity

Non-modifiable
• Age, gender, obesity • Pre-existing liver or chronic renal disease • Renal hypoperfusion • Sepsis
Modifiable
• Choice of aminoglycosides (inherent nephrotoxic potential). • Drug dose per day, drug interval, duration of therapy. • Volume depletion (most important clinically). • Hypokalemia and hypomagnesaemia. • Metabolic acidosis. • Concurrent drug administration (synergism)—other nephrotoxic agents such as amphotericin B, cephalothin, vancomycin, cisplatin, furosemide, calcium channel blockers, radiocontrast agents, cyclosporine (interactive nephrotoxicity).

Table 7.6: Approach to prevention of aminoglycosides nephrotoxicity

1. Choice of aminoglycosides.
2. Dosing; as per level of GFR, monitoring of serum levels.
3. Monitor renal function (creatinine levels every 2-3 days or more.
4. Frequently depending on renal function.
5. Single daily dosing (less nephrotoxic with no loss efficacy, post-antibiotic effect and concentration dependent killing). Dose to be administered during the early afternoon.
6. Modifying 'correctable' factors (mentioned in Table 7.4).
7. Avoiding interactive/synergistic nephrotoxic combinations.

The nephrotoxic potential of various aminoglycosides differs with gentamicin being the most toxic, followed by tobramycin, amikacin, netilmicin and streptomycin. In an attempt to choose the correct dose or drug internal, monitoring of drug levels would seem a rational approach. With rising creatinine aminoglycosides therapy may need to be replaced by appropriate but non-nephrotoxic antibiotics. Other antibiotics that need to be dealt with is the antifungal antibiotic amphotericin B.

The adverse effects are related to the daily dose, duration of therapy, pre-existent renal disease (15.4 fold increase in toxicity), renal hypoperfusion, sodium depletion and concomitant drug exposure (diuretics-12.5 fold increase, aminoglycosides, cisplatin, radiocontrast agents and cyclosporine). Daily dose is an important factor with increased nephrotoxicity associated with increasing daily dose (risk increase 1.8 fold with 0.1 mg/kg increase in dose).

Other antibiotics such as beta lactams, vancomycin and sulfonamides exert their inmate nephrotoxic potentials especially when in combination with other nephrotoxic agents.

Radiocontrast Media

Radiocontrast media induced injury constitutes the third leading use of hospital-acquired acute renal failure. Nephrotoxicity is rare in patients with normal renal function (<1%) and hence it is not unexpected that the most important clinical risk factor for nephrotoxicity is a pre-existing, often unrecognized renal insufficiency. In addition to pre-existent renal disease, age, male gender, dehydration/volume depletion, congestive heart failure, proteinuria, abnormal liver function, hyperuricemia, diabetes mellitus with renal insufficiency, multiple myeloma (precipitation of light chains in an intratubular location due to dehydration and intratubular calcium), cardiovascular disease, hypertension, renal transplantation, large doses of radiocontrast or repeated studies, type of contrast media (ionic or non-ionic), injection site-intra-arterial vs intravenous and concomitant exposure to other nephrotoxic agents are risk factors for nephrotoxicity.

Angiotensin Converting Enzyme (ACE) inhibitors and Angiotensin II Receptor Blockers (ARBs)

Although used for renal protection the ACE inhibitors and the ARBs albeit to a lesser degree may produce renal failure. The occurrence of functional acute renal failure correlates with a loss of post-glomerular efferent arteriolar vascular tone and is usually reversible with drug withdrawal.

Prevention of ACEI and ARB induced nephrotoxicity is dependent on anticipation of its occurrence depending on the existence of risk recognition of risk factors. Vigilant monitoring and volume management are important to this. "Diuretic holiday" may be prescribed, especially in the first few days after ACEI therapy initiation. Another option is the initiation of therapy with a short acting ACEI like captopril, titrating the dose upward in response to blood pressure and renal function. With renal function stable, switch to a long acting ACE inhibitor. The initial days after ACEI (or ARB) therapy is initiated, there is a need to monitor renal function, weekly for the first four week, later monthly and three monthly thereafter. If the creatinine rise is <30% then the therapy could be a beneficial for a better long term outcome. Elevation in creatinine significantly necessitates termination of therapy.

PREVENTION STRATEGIES

Specific certain patients and clinical situations seem to be susceptible to nephrotoxicity. The recognition of the factors that predispose to nephrotoxicity of drugs would enable attempts at limiting or preventing the same. Table 7.7 has listed risk factors for drug nephrotoxicity.

The occurrence or even the prevention of drug-related renal disease should be approached with emphasis on the above-mentioned risk factors. The risk factors take into consideration a factor that range from the patient to the drug-related factors and visualizes the potential of drug interactions in the causation or potentiation of nephrotoxicity.

Table 7.7: Risk factors for nephrotoxicity

Patient-related factors
• Age, sex, race • Pre-existent renal disease • Specific disease (diabetes mellitus, multiple myeloma, proteinuria patients, lupus) • Sodium-retaining states (cirrhosis, heart failure, nephrosis) • Dehydration and volume depletion • Acidosis, potassium and magnesium depletion • Hyperuricemia, hyperuricosuria • Sepsis, shock • Renal transplant.
Drug-related factors
• Inherent nephrotoxic potential • Dose • Duration, frequency and form of administration • Repeated exposure.
Drug interactions
• Combined or closely associated use of diagnostic or therapeutic with added or synergistic nephrotoxic potential (*e.g.* Radiocontrast agents, aminoglycosides, NSAIDs, Cisplatin, ACEI).

A sizeable proportion of the patients having chronic tubulointerstitial nephritis and reaching the ESRD could well be related to the consumption of drugs in the patient with pre-existent renal insufficiency a step-wise approach can be helpful in avoiding nephrotoxicity. After recording the history and performing a physical examination, determine the degree of renal insufficiency through laboratory test. Medication review should be followed by choice of a less nephrotoxic agent. Loading doses permit early achievement of therapeutic levels and subsequent maintenance doses (either reduction of dose or the interval extension method). Measurement of levels definitely help, constant reassessment for efficacy as well as toxicity is essential.

To the internists nephrotoxic quarter (NSAIDs, ACEIs radiocontrast media, aminoglycosides), newer drugs especially finding usage in specific situations are being continually added to this list.

CHAPTER EIGHT

Pulmonary ADRs

Pulmonology has established itself as a subspeciality of medicine though a little in developing countries. Drug induced respiratory diseases are becoming quite increasingly apparent as more than 40 commonly used drugs are reported to cause pulmonary parenchymal tissue injury. Drug induced interstitial lung diseases can be acute or chronic. Due to irreversible damage that may result from drugs, treatment for lethal diseases has to be withdrawn prematurely. It is difficult to estimate the true incidence of drug induced pulmonary disease because of the lack of specific markers, histologic findings or diagnostic clinical features and also because of sporadic nature of many of these reactions. Pharmacologic agents that may cause pulmonary parenchymal injury can be classified into 2 groups (Table 8.1). The first group involves cytotoxic drugs and the second non cytotoxic drugs.

Mechanism of Action

The lungs, the only organs in man are exposed to both internal and external insults of various types and have a number of homeostatic mechanisms for maintaining a balance between damaging inflammatory reaction and protective detoxification pathways. Drugs can affect any of these systems resulting in pulmonary injury. Four types of mechanisms have been put forth.

a. Oxidant-Antioxidant System

Drugs such as bleomycin, cyclophosphamide and amiodarone are capable of producing reactive oxygen

Table 8.1: Drugs causing pulmonary damage

Cytotoxic drugs	*Non- Cytotoxic drugs*
1. Antibiotics	1. Antimicrobial Agents
Bleomycin	Nitrofurantoin
Mitomycin	Amphotericin
	Sulfasalazine
2. Alkylating agents	2. Analgesics Aspirin
Busulfan	
Cyclophosphamide	3. Anticonvulsants
Melphalan	Dipheny hydantion
3. Antimetabolites	Carbamazepine
Methotrexate	4. Antiarrhythmics
Azathioprine	Amiodarone
Mercaptopurine	Lidocaine
Cytosine arabinoside	Procainamide
4. Nitrosoureas	5. Beta adrenergic blocker
Carmustine (BCNU)	Practolol
Semustie(MethylCCNU)	Propranolol
Chlorozotocin	Pindolol
5. Miscellaneous	6. Diuretics
Procarbazine	Hydrochlorothiazide
VM-267	7. Opiates
Vinblastine	Heroin
Vindesine	Propoxyphene
	Methadone
	8. Sedatives
	Chlordiazepoxide
	9. Tranquilizers
	Haloperidol
	Fluphenazine
	10. Miscellaneous
	Gold salts
	Penicillamine
	Isoniazid
	Colchicine

species (oxidants) including the superoxide anion, hydrogen peroxide, the hydroxyl radical (OH), singlet oxygen and hypochlorous acid (HOCL). These oxidants can cause autologous cytotoxicity, unless they are neutralized by antioxidants such as superoxide dismutase (SOD), catalase, glutathione peroxidase, ceruloplasmin and vitamin E. These antioxidant systems are present in virtually every cell in the body. Over production of oxidants by the drugs, thus results in an alteration of normal balance between oxidants and antioxidants resulting in pulmonary toxicity. Oxidant damage can stimulate the immune system and attract neutrophils with protease activity.

b. Immunologic System

Normal resident pulmonary cells are alveolar macrophage and lymphocytes. Drugs can activate resident pulmonary cells resulting in attracting and activating peripheral inflammatory cells such as polymorphonuclear neutrophils (PMN), eosinophils and monocytes. These activated cells liberate cytotoxic mediators. Experimental pulmonary fibrosis induced by agents such as bleomycin, paraquat, N-nitroso-N-methylurethane etc. had shown that fibrosis of the alveolar wall first requires "injury" to the alveolar wall, that is, damage to the existing cells and matrix, comprising the lung parenchyma. More of the injury results from the effector processes of these cell types comprising alveolitis. Bronchoalveolar lavage (BAL) studies have demonstrated increased numbers of induced pulmonary injury. A lymphocytic alveolitis In the BAL has been demonstrated in lung damaged due to bleomycin, methotrexate, gold salts, amiodarone and nitrofurantoin. Lung eosinophilia has been reported in lung diseases due to bleomycin, procarbazine nitrofurantoin, gold etc. The relative potency of the effector cells in regard to their ability to injure the alveolar wall is probably, in descending order, neutrophils, alveolar macrophages, eosinophils and lymphocytes. If the damage is sufficient such that normal alveolar architecture cannot be reestablished, a secondary form of "repair", i.e. replacement of the normal parenchyma by fibroblasts and their products takes over. Activated alveolar macrophages release chemotactants for neutrophils. Leukotriene B, interleukin (IL)-1, possible interleukin, oxidants and a variety of growth signals for mesenchymal cells including platelet derived growth factor (PDGF-B) fibronectin (FN) insulin like growth factor 1 (IGF-1), transforming growth factor beta (TGF-B) and tumour necrosis factor (TNF). Macrophage derived growth factors are shown in figure. Neutrophils release oxidants and potent proteinases such as collagenase and neutrophil elastase. Eosinophils liberate oxidants, collagenase and a variety of other agents such as major basic protein. Lymphocytes release interleukin, migration inhibition factor, monocytes chemotactic factor and oxidants.

Fibronectin and alveolar macrophage derived growth factors (AMDGF), the mediators released by alveolar macrophages play an important role in fibrosis. Fibronectin (FN) recruits fibroblasts to the area of injury. Fibroblast numbers expand as a result of mediators released by macrophages. FN attaches fibroblasts to matrix which is made up of type 1 and type HI collagen. FN also acts as a "competence factor" to move fibroblasts through the early phases of the GI portion of the cell cycle (GI is the earliest phase of the cell proliferation cycle and precedes DNA synthesis). AMDGF acts as a growth factor and in the presence of the "competence factor" (FN) induces fibroblasts to move, through the late stages of GI and proliferate. This ultimately leads to fibrosis by replacement of normal parenchymal cells and matrix by fibroblasts and fibroblast products. However, macrophages are also capable of arresting fibrotic response by releasing two cytokines, TNF-a and IL. They interact synergistically to augment production of prostaglandin (PG) which is a powerful second messenger that inhibits fibroblast proliferation.

c. Proteolytic System

Proteolytic enzymes, particularly elastase are produced by polymorphonuclear leukocytes and alveolar macrophages. There are a number of antiprotease systems in the lower respiratory tract, the most important being the alpha protease inhibitor. Reactive oxygen radicals released by drugs such as bleomycin and cyclophosphamide can inactivate alpha-protease inhibitor resulting in enhanced activity of proteolytic enzymes.

d. Central Nervous System (CNS)

A variety of CNS insults can cause neurogenic pulmonary edema in which there will be an increased capillary protein leak. This may suggest that pulmonary capillary permeability may be, in part, controlled by the central nervous system. Several drugs such as opiates, major tranquilizers, salicylate and methotrexate may cause pulmonary oedema through their effect on CNS. Presence of plentiful opiate receptors near the medullary respiratory centre may support for neural influences in the development of pulmonary oedema.

RISK FACTORS

Pulmonary involvement under the effect of drug therapy depends on certain risk factors, which possibly predispose or precipitate. Risk factors predisposing to development of drug induced pulmonary disease are given in Table 8.2. These include the drug dosage which may affect the lungs due to cumulative effect e.g. bleomycin, amiodarone etc. or the unit dose may cause the pulmonary disease as seen with many drugs like amiodarone, chlordiazepoxide, colchicine, haloperidol, imipramine etc. Apart from drug dosage, the frequency of drug administration as with methotrexate and the route of dispensing the drug as with bleomycin, also form important risk factors in developing drug induced pulmonary disease.

Associated radiotherapy with bleomycin, mitomycin, busulfan and oxygen therapy alongwith cyclophosphamide, nitrofurantoin and mitomycin predispose to pulmonary involvement. Associated other drug therapy like bleomycin, BCNU, vinca alkaloids etc., other preexisting pulmonary disease with BCNU, amiodarone, other systemic illness like renal failure with bleomycin, blood transfusions with amphotericin and mitomycin, pulmonary angiography with amiodarone, steroid therapy with methotrexate may predispose to drug induced pulmonary involvement.

Table 8.2: Risk factors for pulmonary toxicity

Risk factor	*Drugs implicated*
1. **Dose**	
a. Cumulative dose	Bleomycin, Carmustine (BCNU), Amiodarone
b. Unit dose	Amiodarone, Heroin, methadone, Ethcholorvynol, Colchicine, Imipramine
2. **Dispensing**	
a. Route of administration	Bleomycin
b. Freqtuency of administration	Methotrexate
3. **Mother Modes**	
a. Oxygen therapy	Bleomycin, Mitomycin, Cyclophosphamide, Nitrofurantoin
b. Radio therapy	Bleomycin, Busulfan, Mitomycin
	Bleomycin, BCNU, Cyclophosphamide.
4. **Anti-cancer drugs**	Mitomycin, Methotrexate, Vinca alkaloids
5. **Other factors**	
a. Age	Bleomycin
b. Previous pulmonary diseases	BCNU, Amiodarone
c. Blood component transfusions	Mitomycin, Amphotericin
d. Renal failure	Bleomycin
e. Steroid tapering or adrenalectomy	Methotrexate
f. Pulmonary angiography	Amiodarone

Clinical Manifestations

Symptoms

- Cough.
- Wheezing.
- Shortness of breath.
- Chest pain.
- Bloody sputum.
- Fever.

Symptoms may vary.

Signs and Tests

- Abnormal breath sounds revealed by a physical examination with a stethoscope.
- Chest X-ray.
- Chest CT scan.
- CBC with differential.
- Bronchoscopy.
- Thoracentesis if pleural effusion is present.
- Rarely, difficult to diagnose cases may require lung biopsy.

Six distinct syndromes have been described clinically.

1. **Pneumonitis/fibrosis**: Drugs causing pneumonitis/ fibrosis are shown in Table 8.3. Symptoms begin insidiously, progressing over several weeks to months. Symptoms include non-productive cough, dyspnoea on exertion, fatigue and malaise. Significant weight loss can also occur. Bi-basilar end-expiratory crackles can be heard on auscultation. Clubbing may be present. The chest radiograph show bilateral reticular infiltrates. Occasionally chest radiograph is initially normal, even in the presence of pulmonary symptoms and physiologic abnormalities. Pulmonary function may show a restrictive ventilatory defect with a reduced diffusing capacity. In general, most patients show some residual pulmonary impairment despite appropriate treatment which include

Table 8.3: Drugs causing pneumonitis/firbositis

Chemotherapeutic agents for cancer
Bleomycin
Mitomycin
Busulfan
Cyclophosphamide
Melphalan
Carmustine (BCNU)
Semustine (Methyl CCNU)
Lomustine (CCNU)
Chlorozotocin
Methotrexate

discontinuation of the offending drug and institution of corticosteroids. We don't really know whether steroids help as there are no studies, but there is little to lose by trying them.

2. **Hypersensitivity Pneumonitis (Eosinophilic pulmonary infiltration): Drugs** that cause hypersensitivity pneumonitis (HP) are shown in Table 8.4. HP is characterised by a subacute onset (within hours to days) of dyspnoea, non-productive cough, chills, myalgia, fever and headache. Skin rash may be present in 50% of patients. Auscultation may reveal crackles. 40% of patients will have peripheral eosinophilia. There may be signs of hepatitis in a few cases. The chest radiograph shows diffuse acinar infiltrates, pleural effusions are more common than those of pneumonitis. Pulmonary function shows restriction with mildly reduced diffusing capacity. Lung biopsy may show interstitial and airway eosinophilia with a paucity of fibrosis. Virtually all patients, except those due to methotrexate, recover with few residual pulmonary dysfunctions. Treatment includes withdrawal of the drug and institution of corticosteroids.

Table 8.4: Drugs causing hypersensitivity pneumonitis

Nitrofurantoin
Naproxen
Procarbazine
Paraminosalicyclic acid
Penicillin
Pyrimethamine
Sulfasalazine

3. **Non-Cardiogenic pulmonary oedema:** Symptoms occur acutely (over minutes to hours) and usually are associated with overdose of the offending agents. Drugs that cause non-cardiogenic pulmonary oedema are given in Table 8.5. Prognosis is variable and generally better than other causes of non-cardiogenic pulmonary oedema on removal of the offending agents.
4. **Bronchiolitis obleterans:** This rare complication is usually due to three drugs namely gold salts,

Table 8.5 : Drugs causing non-cardiogenic pulmonary oedema

Chemotherapeutic
Cyclophosphamide
Cytosine arabinoside
Mitomycine
Methtrexate
VM-26
Other drugs
Amphotericin
Chlordiazepoxide
Colchicine
Ethchlorvynol
Heroin
Haloperidon
Isoxsuprine
Imipramine
Lidocaine
Methadone
Propoxyphene
Ritodrine
Terbutaline

sulfasalazine and penicillamine. The underlying disease particularly rheumatoid arthritis can cause similar pulmonary pathology in the absence of drugs. Clinical symptoms include insidious onset of cough dyspnoea and weight loss. Chest radiographs may be normal or show localized infiltrate. Pulmonary function test shows an obstructive ventilatory defect. Histology shows areas of inflammation surrounding bronchioles resulting in their obliteration. In a proportion of patients especially due to sulfasalazine and penicillamine, a significant alveolitis is present. Prognosis of this condition is poor. Despite corticosteroid treatment and discontinuation of drugs the offending agents, residual pulmonary abnormalities will be persisting.

5. **Pulmonary renal syndrome:** This is a rare complication of penicillamine treatment. Clinical presentation includes hemoptysis, dyspnoea, pleuritic chest pain and uremia. Chest radiographic abnormalities include diffuse acinar, reticular or confluent large round

densities. Lung histology shows pulmonary haemorrhage and haemosiderin laden macrophages. Although similar to Good Pasture's syndrome, there is no typical linear pattern of basement membrane immunoglobulin deposition. Treatment includes immunosuppression and plasmapheresis.

6. **Airways obstruction:** Airways obstruction presenting as cough, chest and asthma has been observed with drugs like beta blockers, non-steroidal anti-inflammatory drugs, prostaglandin F_2a and ACE inhibitors. This may happen with laxatives and antidepressants. Also asthma may occur with selective beta blockers which need to be contraindicated in asthma patients.

SCREENING TESTS

1. **Diffusing capacity for carbon monoxide (TLCO):** TLCO appears to be a sensitive, but relatively non-specific test as a predictor of drug induced pneumonitis especially in bleomycin or amiodarone-induced pneumonitis. Patients who never develop clinical disease had also shown a reduced TLCO. It is less helpful if only one reading is available after the patient has lung disease. Baseline reading is always helpful.
2. **Lung volumes:** A reduction in lung volumes is a restrictive ventilatory defect, appears to be a specific test, but is not very sensitive. Patients with lung disease have rarely shown normal lung volumes. Specificity is less since a wide variety of lung diseases do produce reduction in lung volumes.
3. **Computed tomographic (CT) scanning:** The detection of fibrosis by CT scanning has been correlated with lung volume measurements. CT abnormalities were detected in patients with normal chest radiographs. However, CT may not differentiate reversible pneumonitis from irreversible fibrosis. CT may prove to be sensitive and specific test in predicting development of drug induced lung disease, slightly more sensitive than chest radiographer but rarely indicated.

4. **Chest radiographs:** Chest radiographs are both nonspecific and insensitive in pulmonary disease. An abnormal chest radiograph is a late manifestation of drug induced lung disease.
5. **Gallium scanning:** Gallium scanning is not specific. However, positive gallium scans i.e. uptake of gallium-67 in area of acute inflammation, in the absence of abnormal chest radiographs have been reported in drug induced lung diseases. However, there are no proper studies to evaluate gallium scanning in drug induced disease.
6. **Soluble mediators:** Soluble mediators such as serum angiotensin converting enzyme have been described in all patients receiving bleomycin, but most of them do not develop pulmonary fibrosis. This is a fertile field for future research in drug induced lung disease.

Treatment

Treatment consists mainly of discontinuing the offending drug immediately, and beginning supportive management of the symptoms. For instance, you may need inhaler therapy and oxygen until the drug induced lung disease improves. Challenge tests (reintroducing the suspected medication to see if symptoms recur) are rarely performed. Steroid therapy such as prednisone, to quickly reverse the lung inflammation caused by the offending drug, is sometimes used.

Acute episodes usually resolve within 48-72 hours after the medication has been discontinued, but chronic syndromes may take longer to resolve. Some drug induced lung diseases such as pulmonary fibrosis may never resolve.

To conclude, one can precisely say that no organ system in the body functions in an isolation. And lungs are no exception to this rule. Rather aerosol therapy can cause cardiac failure, myocardial fibrosis, left ventricular dysfunction or pericarditis and propranolol, amiodarone, thiazides, practolol hydralazine, aspirin etc. can cause bronchospasm, alveolitis, pulmonary oedema, pleural fibrosis, lupus syndrome and bronchial asthma respectively. So, it is always wise to use the minimum and most appropriate drugs and keep in mind the interface and the possible drug reactions in the lungs so as to act urgently to remove the offending agents and institute the therapy.

CHAPTER NINE

Endocrinal ADRs

Majority of drug induced endocrine disturbances are type A reactions and hence are generally preventable and reversible. Type B reactions are a few, e.g. β-cell cytotoxicity of pentamidine, thyroid autoimmunity induced by iodides and lithium. Drug induced endocrinopathies can be divided into two:

a. Drugs used for endocrinal disorders inducing endocrinopathies.
b. Drugs used for Non-endocrine disorders inducing endocrinopathies.

Drug inducing endocrinopathies disorders pose a very common differential diagnose and hence knowledge of drug effect is very important to avoid unnecessary expensive laboratory tests and treatment. Most of these adverse effects are reversible by reduction or modification of therapy. Since most of them are type A effects.

Drugs produce adverse effects on the endocrine system by their pharmacokinetic or pharmacodynamic properties. The former includes (a) interference in absorption and bioavailability (e.g. cholestyramine and soya flour products interfere with T4 absorption) and (b) displacement from binding proteins (e.g. NSAIDs induced displacement of T4 and T3 from TBG). The pharmacodynamic effects of drugs on the endocrine system include those on hormone synthesis, transport, action and metabolic clearance brought about by one or more of the following:

i. Alteration in electrolyte balance which in turn influences hormone secretion or action (e.g.

decrease in insulin release by thiazides through hypokalemia).

ii. Alteration in transmembrane ion fluxes (e.g. effect of calcium channel blockers on insulin release from pancreatic cells).

iii. Effect on neurotransmitters that modulate hormone secretion and release (e.g. β-blockers effect on insulin, dopaminergic antagonists on prolactin secretion).

iv. Modification in signal transduction resetting of homeostatic mechanism (e.g. effect of lithium on parathormone secretion).

v. Inhibition of key enzymes involved in hormone synthesis (e.g. effect of ketoconazole on cortisol and androgen biosynthesis by inhibiting cytochrome P_{450} enzymes plasma, augmentation in TBG, CBG concentration by estrogens).

vi. Agonistic action through structural similarities with endogenous ligands (e.g. synthetic glucocorticoids action at hormone-receptor level, glucocorticoids and OCs on insulin action).

vii. Alteration in degradative enzymes leading to change in hormone clearance (e.g. Rifampicin, phenobarbitone on thyroxin and cortisol).

The effect of drugs on the endocrine system are:

1. Usually duration and dose related.
2. The induced laboratory abnormalities need to be distinguished from clinically evident side effects.
3. Two or more drugs may have additive or synergistic action in bringing about the undesirable effect and conversely one drug can act through multiple mechanisms.
4. The same drug may have entirely opposite actions on some variable depending on patient characteristics, underlying the disease etc. (e.g. β-blockers effect on glucose homeostasis, effect of iodine and iodine containing drugs on thyroid status).

Even though some of the adverse effects of drugs have been converted to therapeutic advantage (e.g. antiandrogenic property of spironolactone in hirsutism, inhibition of steroidogenesis by ketoconazole in Cushing's syndrome), in majority of instances they endanger morbidity, confusion with endocrine hypo or hyper function states and costly and time consuming investigations. Some adverse effects are potentially life threatening e.g. drug induced hypoglycemia, exogenous glucocorticoids induced HPA axis suppression. Hence a thorough knowledge of adverse endocrine effect of drugs is desirable.

ADVERSE EFFECTS

1. EFFECTS ON GLUCOSE TOLERANCE

Hyperglycemia

Several drugs induce glucose intolerance in non-diabetics and worsen control in diabetics by altering insulin secretion and/or insulin action at various levels. Thiazides diuretics are one of the major drugs that produce hyperglycemia. This effect is dose related. A 30% incidence of glucose intolerance in hypertensive patients receiving thiazides has been reported. Decreased insulin secretion because of hypokalemia appears to be the major mechanism as potassium supplementation improves their glycemic status. Other mechanisms include elevated free fatty acids impairing insulin action, direct cytotoxic effect of thiazides, increased hepatic glucose output, enhanced catecholamine secretion and action and increased glucagons secretion. Loop diuretics (furosemide and ethacrynic acid) and potassium sparing diuretics have less adverse effect on glucose tolerance. Expectedly chlorthalidone therapy is associated with higher incidence and higher grade glucose intolerance than hydrochlorothiazide and indapamide is devoid of any glucose intolerant effect.

The lipophilic non selective β-blockers (e.g. propranolol) inhibit insulin release and enhance hepatic glucose production. Though marked hyperglycemia is uncommon, hyperosmolar coma has been precipitated by these drugs in a few instances. Calcium channel blockers can reduce insulin secretion as insulin release is dependent on an increase in cystolic calcium. However no consistent adverse clinical effect has been noted with nifedipine. Verapamil has been noted to have contradictory effects, improvement as well as worsening of glucose tolerance in different studies. The potential adverse effects on insulin secretion seem to be balanced by the vasodilatory property of these agents that improves insulin delivery to tissues. Still these agents do not have clinically significant effects on glucose metabolism.

Though clonidine by its alpha-2 agonistic property is expected to reduce insulin secretion, it is not clinically significant in most instances. Cyclosporine has a dose-dependent hyperglycemic effect by its direct cytotoxic effect and questionable effect on insulin action. This is of relevance since after pancreatic transplantation, the incidence of persisting insulin requirement is higher among patients receiving cyclosporine than those receiving azathioprine.

Phenytoin leads to hypoinsulinemia secondary to impaired insulin release. Though significant impairment of glucose tolerance is not found, cases of hyperosmolar coma have been noted occasionally. Glucocorticoids lead to insulin resistance at receptor and post receptor levels as well as increase gluconeogenesis and hyperglucagonemia. They can unmask underlying glucose intolerance or precipitate hyperosmolar coma in already diabetic patients. This effect is dose related and usually due to systemic use of these drugs though potent topical steroids used over large surface area and over prolonged duration can also produce glucose intolerance. Glucocorticoids that are oxygenated at 11 and 17 positions (e.g. hydrocortisone) and those which have 1, 2 double bond in A ring (prednisone and prednisolone) have the most diabetogenic effects. ACTH has similar effect. Though mineralocorticoids do not directly influence carbohydrate metabolism, they can reduce insulin secretion through hypokalemia.

The adverse effects of oral contraceptives on glucose tolerance are largely due to the progestogen component especially the 19-nortestosterone derivatives. Though estrogens increase growth hormone and cortisol and cortisol induced increase in hepatic gluconeognesis has been postulated to increase glucose intolerance. Low dose ethinyl estradiol formulations and conjugated estrogens have negligible effects on glucose tolerance. Interestingly low dose transdermal 17-beta estradiol in post menopausal women improves glucose tolerance by increasing hepatic insulin clearance. The new triphasic oral contraceptives containing levonorgesterol and ehtinyl estradiol have minimal effect on carbohydrate metabolism. Hence, diabetes has not been shown to be an important contraindication to hormonal contraception.

Nicotinic acid is most likely to induce severe hyperglycemia in patients with established glucose intolerance or in those receiving other diabetogenic medications through impairment of insulin action as well as release. Beta adrenergic agonists can increase plasma glucose values if enhanced glycogenolysis and lipolysis predominate despite increased insulin secretion. Large dose of I.V. salbutamol has been known to induce diabetic ketoacidosis (DKA). Oral terbutaline and to a lesser extent ritodrine also cause glucose intolerance. Other drugs implicated occasionally in diabetogenesis are: L-asparaginase, isoniazid, morphine, doxapram, dopamine and its analogues dapsone, nalidixic acid, rifampicin, indomethacin, chlordiazepoxide and possibly amiodarone.

Hypoglycemia

Hypoglycemia is a potentially life threatening complication caused by some drugs, which may produce this effect *de novo* but more commonly, by enhancing the hypoglycemic effect of insulin or oral hypoglycemic agents. Prompt recognition is important not only from management point of view, but also to prevent irreversible brain damage, and also lo avoid costly and time consuming investigations for rarer disorders like insulinoma.

Drugs causing hypoglycemia do so by either increasing insulin secretion, potentiating insulin action or by decreasing hepatic gluconeognesis. Though salicylates are implicated as a major cause of hypoglycemia in children in case of over dose, aspirin rarely causes hypoglycemia in healthy adults. It is reported to reduce insulin requirement in IDDM patients and potentiate hypoglycemic action of sulfonylureas in NIDDM subjects. The effects are usually seen with daily doses of 4-6 gms that are used in rheumatoid arthritis. The mechanisms include reduced insulin clearance, increased insulin secretion, reduction of gluconeognesis and enhancement of peripheral glucose utilization. Sulfamethoxazole used alone or in combination with sulfonylureas induce hypoglycemia especially in patients with renal failure by increasing insulin secretion, due to their structural similarity to sulfonylureas. Non selective beta blockers can cause severe hypoglycemia in both diabetic and non diabetic patients especially in the former with concomitant insulin or oral antidiabetic (OADs) use. The mechanisms contributing to hypoglycemia include enhancement of insulin action, inhibition of lipolysis and glycogenolysis and glucagon mediated gluconeognesis. In addition the adrenergic symptoms of hypoglycemia may be masked, though sweating is unimpaired, since it is mediated by post ganglionic cholinergic fibers. The use of cardio selective beta blockers may lessen the chances of hypoglycemia in high risk patients.

Quinine has been well documented to cause profound hypoglycemia during treatment of falciparum malaria. In addition to possible excess glucose consumption by the parasitized RBCs, the other mechanisms contributing to hypoglycemia include enhanced insulin release by direct action on β cells and inhibition of hepatic gluconeognesis. Octreotide has been found to be useful in reversing hypoglycemia in refractory cases.

β_2 adrenergic agonists (e.g. salbutamol) have been reported to cause prolonged hypoglycemia in both the mother and infant when used as tocolytic agents. This effect is mediated through increased insulin secretion. Disopyramide, a quinidine like agent, causes marked fasting hypoglycemia especially in patients with hepatic or renal disease or in elderly. The mechanisms are similar to that of quinine. Monoamine oxidase inhibitors cause hypoglycemia through their β-cytotoxic effect. ACE inhibitors can cause hypoglycemia and lead to decrease in insulin or sulfonylurea requirement in diabetic patients. This effect is attributed to increase in plasma bradykinin levels that enhance insulin sensitivity. Other drugs implicated in causing hypoglycemia include lidocaine, lithium, quinidine, dextropropoxyphene (in renal failure), temafloxacillin, a newer quinolone antibiotics and tetracyclines.

Drug Causing Hypoglycemia As Well As Hyperglycemia

Pentamidine, a biguanide derivative is used in treatment of antimony resistant Kala-azar and pneumnocystis carinii pneumonia in AIDS patients has a biphasic effect on blood glucose similar to other β cytotoxic agents (streptozotocin and alloxan). Hypoglycemia is noted in 27% of patients receiving petamidine for pneumocystis infection. The major mechanism is cytotoxic effect on pancreatic cells leading to early cytolytic release of insulin followed by diabetes. An extra pancreatic effect similar to biguanide has also been reported. Pentamidine isethionate is apparently less than pentamidine mesylate.

β blockers cause hyperglycemia in subjects with underlying glucose intolerance while causing hypoglycemia in diabetics on insulin or OADs though the converse may also occur. This apparent paradox is due to factors such as dose, nutritional state, concomitant medications, severity of underlying-illness and β cell reserve. β2 agonists similarly have effect on plasma glucose depending on which of their effect is predominating (insulin secretagogue vs lipolytic, glycogenolytic actions). While interpreting drug effects it is also important to bear in mind the role of concomitant alcohol ingestion, as acutely it is known to cause hypoglycemia and on chronic use worsens glucose intolerance.

2. ADVERSE DRUG EFFECTS ON THYROID FUNCTION

Drugs alter thyroid function either by affecting thyroid hormone biosynthesis or by modulating their transport, cellular uptake and degradation. While the former is responsible for clinical hypo or hyperfunction of the gland, the latter mechanisms account, for alterations in various thyroid function tests. The same drug may act at multiple levels and have varying consequences. Other variables like patient characteristics, underlying disease, iodine intake etc. may influence the action.

Drug induced alterations of thyroid function may result in:

a. Laboratory abnormalities which are not clinically significant.
b. Dual effects on thyroid function, hyper or hypothyroidism.
c. Goiter with or without hypothyroidism.

a. Drug Causing Alterations in Thyroid Function Tests

Drug Altering Binding of Thyroid Hormones in Plasma

Drugs which increase thyroglobulin (TBG) synthesis (e.g. 5-fluorouracil) or decrease its clearance by glycosylation (e.g. estrogens) increase total T4 and T5 as a homeostatic consequence of maintaining normal free hormone concentrations. Conversely, drugs that decrease TBG synthesis (androgens, danazol, anabolic steroids, glucocorticoids and L-asparaginase) decrease total T4 and T3, but free T4 and T3 are maintained at normal levels. NSAIDs (aspirin, diclofenac and mefenamic acid) and heavy doses of furosemide used in venal failure displace T4 and T3 from TBG leading to increase in total hormone levels. Heparin induced rise in free T4 is due to increased free fatty acids that inhibit T4 binding to TBG. This can be offset by inhibitors of lipolysis. The clinical consequences of alteration in T3 and T4 binding are negligible, since no compound provokes a sufficiently severe and prolonged elevation in free hormone. It is still relevant to know these facts to avoid misinterpretation of laboratory results.

Drugs Altering Cellular Uptake of Thyroid Hormones

Phenytoin has been shown to bind to T3 receptors in the pituitary and has an agonistic action in suppressing TSH, leading to low T4 and T3. The clinical consequence of this is however negligible. Amiodarone competes with T5 for binding to pituitary receptors and stimulates TSH release. Similar anti-T3 actions are proposed to be the basis for its antiarrhythmic effect. No clinical consequence has been reported for its effect on TSH.

Drug Inducing Hepatic Microsomal Enzymes

Phenobarbital, phenytoin, carbamazepine and rifampicin induce hepatic microsomal enzymes and there by lead to increase in T4 catabolism and clearance. These drugs reduce T4 but T3 generally is less affected. TSH usually remains normal. Clinically no sign of hypothyroidism is evident in otherwise healthy individuals taking these drugs, but hypothyroids receiving exogenous T4, may require higher dose to maintain euthyroid status.

Drug Affecting Tests of Hypothalamic Pituitary Thyroid axis

TSH response to TRH is augmented by estrogens and theophylline and reduced by glucocorticoids, long term treatment with L-dopa and infusions of dopamine in acute setting, bur these drugs do not cause any clinical thyroid dysfunction.

b. Drugs that cause both Hyper and Hyperthyroidism

Iodine and iodine containing drugs used in therapy and radiographic contrast media (Table 9.1) induce thyroid dysfunctions. Most of those are water soluble with high metabolic clearance. Hence, a prolonged use of the drug in a setting of defective auto-regulation of the thyroid is necessary to have the adverse effect. Route of administration is not important; as both vaginal douching with providone iodine as well as administration of iodinated glycerol orally, are equally reported to cause adverse effects.

Table 9.1: Common iodine containing formulations

Preparation	Iodine content
Oral	
Iodinised glycerol (organ id in)	25 mg/ml
SSKI	47 mg/ml
Lugol's solution	7.8 mg/drop
Amiodarone	75 mg/20 mg tablet
Radiographic	
Diatrizoate (Renografm-60)	290 mg/ml
Lopanoate (Telepaque)	335 mg/500 mg tablet
Lothalamate (Angioconrary)	480 mg/ml
Lopadimol (Isovue - 370)	370mg/ml
Topical	
Clioquinol (vitbrm)	12.5 mg/g
Povidonc-iodine (Betadine]	10 mg/ml
Tincture of iodine	20 mg/ml

Transport of excess iodine into thyroid leads to a block in organification and coupling reactions (Wolf Chaikoff effect). This effect is transient since escape occurs once further iodide transport in to thyroid is inhibited by autoregulatory mechanism. The other effect of excess intrathyroidal iodine is retardation of hormone release through an inhibition of proteolytic release of iodothyronines from thyroglobulin. This effect is also transient like the Wolf-Chaikoff effect, lasting for only a few days.

The pathologic consequences of iodine excess will ensue either because of defective autoregulatory leading to prolonged Wolf-Chaikoff effect or absent autoregulation due to foci of autonomicity in the thyroid. Defective autoregulation leads to sustained inhibition of hormone synthesis and release with subsequent TSH rise, goiter and exacerbation of hypothyroid. This is found in fetal and neonatal thyroid, Hashimoto's thyroiditis, radioiodine or surgically treated Graves' hyperthyroidism, cystic fibrosis, concomitant administration of lithium and sulfonamides. For this reason iodine administration to the mother is contraindicated during pregnancy to avoid fetal goiter and hypothyroidism. Iodine induced goiter and hypothyroidism are usually self limited and subside when excess iodine supply is discontinued. Iodine however can perpetuate thyroid dysfunction indirectly by inducing thyroid autoimmunity.

When autoregulation is absent as in multinodular goiter with foci of autonomicity, iodine administration leads to sustained increase in hormone synthesis and secretion causing thyrotoxicosis (Jod Basedow phenomenon). This is attributed to unmasking of autonomous foci which were dormant. This form of thyrotoxicosis is characterized by decreased radio active iodine uptake and normal or increased T4:T3 ratio. This is a self-limited phenomenon abating after stopping iodine. It can be rapidly alleviated by administration of potassium percholate, an inhibitor of iodine transport.

The antiarrhythmics drug amiodarone contains 37.5% iodine weight by weight. In addition to inhibiting peripheral conversion of T4 to T3 it has effects on thyroid hormone synthesis and secretion through its iodine content. Because of its propensity to be stored in adipose tissue with a slow metabolic disposal its effect can continue for several months after the drugs is withdrawn. The incidence of hyperthyroidism in patients on chronic amiodarone therapy ranges from 0-12% with a mean of 2%. It positively correlates with the duration of therapy and the age of the patient population. Amiodarone induced thyrotoxicosis is characteristically associated with elevated T4:T3 ratio. In view of its iodine content, amiodarone can also induce hypothyroidism (4% in one series after 2-5 years use) especially in the setting of underlying autoimmune thyroid disease.

Drugs Causing Goiter With or Without Hypothyroidism

Drugs interfering with thyroid hormone biosynthesis and release at various steps can induce goiter with or without hypothyroidism (Table 9.2). The most notable of them is lithium, its primary effect being inhibition of hormone release. An additional effect proposed is impairment of hormone synthesis by inhibitory action on TSH, though on long term administration it is overridden by decreased T4 and T3 synthesis leading to increase in iodine uptake and goiter formation. The prevalence of goiter in patients on long term lithium use (manic depressive psychosis) is estimated to be around 1% though individual series have reported higher percentages; hypothyroidism is seen in 2-15% of patients. Though some suggestions are available regarding the role of concomitantly present or lithium induced auto immune thyroid disease in the pathogenesis of hypothyroidism in most instances the hypothyroid state is reversible on discontinuation of the drug. Patient on lithium therapy should have thyroid function tests before they start therapy and during periodic follow-ups. Concomitant iodine administration is to be avoided since they act synergistically to induce hypothyroidism.

The other drugs which inhibit organification and hence are goiterogenic include aminoglutethimide, phenylbutazone, sulfonamides, acetazolamide and sulfonylureas though the effect of the latter group of drugs has been questioned by some studies. Ethionamide, cyclophosphamide and pentazocin have been reported to cause hypothyroidism in isolated instances.

3. ADVERSE DRUG EFFECTS ON ADRENOCORTICAL FUNCTION

Drug induced Cushing's Syndrome and HPA Axis Suppression

Exogenous hypocortisolism has many features similar to endogenous hypocortisolism and proper drug history is a must to exclude exogenous glucocorticoids use before embarking upon investigation for Cushing's syndrome. Some clinical features are specific for drug induced Cushing state, namely posterior subcapsular cataract, glaucoma, panniculitis, pancreatitis, aseptic necrosis of femoral head and pseudotumor cerebri (especially when discontinuing the glucocorticoids therapy). The adverse effects are related to potency of the preparation, dose and duration of treatment, though interindividual variations exist. Even though systemic administration is most commonly associated with undesirable effects, these can occur even with topical dermatologic preparation over large surface area especially with occlusive dressing and over prolonged use.

The major adverse effect of exogenous glucocorticoids that is potentiality life threatening is suppression of hypothalamo pituitary adrenocortical axis (HPA) rendering the patients unable to respond to stress when the therapy is stopped. Abrupt cessation of prolonged glucocorticoids therapy is the commonest cause of secondary adrenocortical insufficiency. The degree of HPA axis suppression depends on a number of factors including duration of therapy, time of day of administration, potency, half life of the drug, route of administration, dose and intervals in split dose regimes. Patients who receive glucocorticoids continuously above the physiological replacement doses for more than 2 weeks, have evidence for HPA axis suppression. It has been found that after one year of continuous therapy with supraphysiologic doses, it takes 9 months to a year for recovery of axis. During this recovery period and for an additional 1-2 years the patients needs to be under steroid cover during periods of stress and both the doctors and patient should be alert to this possibility. HPA axis suppression is more profound if the steroid is administered in the evening.

The more potent and long-acting the steroid, the greater is the degree of suppression (e.g. dexamethasone). Though HPA axis suppression is commonly observed with systemic steroid use, it may occur with potent topical applications (dermatologic ophthalmic preparations and retention enemas) for longer duration. Inhalation of steroids when exceed the oral equivalent physiologic dose (Inhaled Beclomethasone 2 puffs given 4 times daily, a dose 400 µg per day, is equivalent to 7.5 mg prednisolone) can also lead to this complication occasionally. Medroxy progesterone and cyproterone acetate can also produce suppression of HPA axis through receptor cross specificity with those of glucocorticoids. These side effects can he substantially reduced by using minimum effective dose, preferably as alternate day therapy and employing effective non-steroidal modalities of treatment when feasible.

Drugs Causing Adrenal Insufficiency

Ketoconazole and other systemically used imidazole agents decrease cortisol biosynthesis by inhibiting the cytochrome P_{450} enzymes, 11-B hydroxylase and 20, 22 desmolase. It is dose related. Additionally, it exerts anti-glucocorticoids effect at receptor level. Clinically hypoadrenocortisolism is rare, but is recorded in patients with deficient adrenal reserve. Etomidate (an imidazole derivative), has similar effects on cortisol biosynthesis, which may last up to 4 days after discontinuation and cause postoperative hypotension. Rifampicin accelerates cortisol catabolism by hepatic microsomal enzyme induction. While this has little impact in normal individuals, it can precipitate adrenal insufficiency in patients with compromised adrenal reserve and may enhance the steroid requirements in patients on replacement therapy. This effect occurs usually within 2 weeks of initiation of therapy. Suramin used in treatment of trypanosomiasis and recently in HIV infection also causes adrenal insufficiency. Heparin and oral anticoagulants may induce acute adrenocortical failure through bilateral adrenal hemorrhages.

Drug Affecting Mineralocorticoids

Secondary hyperaldosteronism with an increase in plasma renin activity (PRA) and aldosterone has been reported with lithium carbonate and gentamicin. Oral contraceptives contribute to hypertension also through the same mechanism. Licorice and carbonoxolone lead to a state of apparent mineralocorticoid excess with suppressed PRA, hypokalemia and hypertension. This is caused by the active principle glycyrrhizin acid that inhibits conversion of cortisol to cortisone in the renal tubules, thereby allowing it to exert its action on the renal tubular mineralocorticoid receptors. Heparin and related polysulfated glycosaminoglycans (Heparinoids) when given for a prolonged period can produce continued suppression of aldosterone synthesis and secretion from the zona glomerulosa.

4. ADVERSE DRUG EFFECTS ON ADRENAL MEDULLA

Withdrawal of clonidine, ingestion of tyramine containing foods along with monoamine oxidase inhibitors and hypoglyeemic reactions concomitant with the use of β blockers are associated with hypertensive crisis simulating pheochromocytoma. Severe and occasionally fatal paroxysms in pheochromocytoma are induced by opiates, histamine, ACTH, saralasin, glucagon, anesthetic agents like halothane, diethylether, cyclopropane, tricyclic antidepressants, methyldopa, guanethidine, bethanidine, debrisoquine and bretylium tosylate. Alpha adrenergic agonists (nasal decongestants) and use of β-blockers without prior alpha blockade also cause severe exacerbations of hypertension in these patients. In addition, many drugs interfere with laboratory tests for confirmation of the diagnosis of pheochromocytoma and hence have to be avoided

5. ADVERSE DRUG EFFECTS ON BONE AND MINERAL METABOLISM

Hypocalcaemia

Long term use of anticonvulsants (phenytoin, phenobarbitone and less often carbamazepine) leads to hypocalcaemia in 20-30% of patients with epilepsy. This is due to a state of functional vitamin D deficiency by accelerated hepatic catabolism due to induction of microsomal enzymes. Vitamin D malabsorption also causes hypocalcaemia. There are a few case reports of hypocalcaemia caused by high dose ketoconazole used in treatment of prostatic cancer by inhibition of 1-hydroxylase and the resultant decrease in 1,25-(OH)2 D3. Parenteral phosphate therapy used previously in treatment of hypocalcaemia is notorious to cause hypocalcaemia. Ibuprofen has been noted lo cause hypocalcaemia in patients with rheumatoid arthritis by inhibition of PTH action. Hyperparathyroidism hypocalcaemia and hypomagnesaemia can occur during treatment of acute leukemia with adriamycin and cytosine arabinoside.

Hypocalcaemia

Ingestion of high doses of vitamin D of its analogs is the major cause of drug induced hypocalcaemia. The toxic dose has wide interindividual variations bur generally exceeds 50,000 units per day. Reversibility is rapid following discontinuance of shorter acting analogues but not so with the long acting natives. Vitamin D sensitivity occurs during post-partum period and in idiopathic hypocalcaemia of infancy and sarcoidosis. Prolonged excessive ingestion of calcium accompanied by systemic antacid therapy (milk-alkali syndrome) is another cause of hypocalcaemia, rarely seen now. Vitamin A intoxication can lead to hypocalcaemia occasionally. Thiazides induced self-limiting hypocalcaemia is significant only in the setting of preexisting disease like hyperparathyroidism. Contracted intravascular volume and increased tubular reabsorption of calcium along with sodium in the proximal segment are contributing factors. Chronic aluminium toxicity due to haemodialysis in chronic renal failure leads lo hypocalcaemia, when vitamin D analogues are used without chelators like desferrioxamine to remove aluminium from the mineralisation front. Rarely symptomatic hypocalcaemia is induced by tamoxifen in patients of breast carcinoma with widespread skeletal metastases. Lithium treatment may lead to hypocalcaemia in 8-21% of patient (13% in a series of patients receiving the drug for a period of 6 years). This is caused by direct stimulation of the parathyroid by lithium and resetting of the calcium-stat at a higher level. Both parathyroid hyperplasia and adenoma have been reported in a few cases but direct causal relationship is difficult to demonstrate.

Lithium also has extra parathyroid effects leading to an increase in intestinal absorption and renal tubular reabsorption of calcium. Though in majority of instances hypocalcaemia is mild and asymptomatic, surveillance for this complication is warranted by pre-therapy calcium estimation followed by annual measurement of serum calcium in patients on chronic lithium therapy.

Osteoporosis

Prolonged exogenous glucocorticoids therapy exceeding 15 mg prednisolone or its equivalent daily leads to varying grades of osteoporosis in most instances. This is due to direct suppression of osteoblastic activity, antianabolic action on bone matrix and negative calcium balance caused by decreased intestinal absorption of calcium and hypercalciuria that account for secondary hyperparathyroidism. The hypogonadal state induced by chronic steroid therapy adds to the problem. Though trabecular bone of spine is most commonly affected, fractures of femoral necks, ribs and long bones are also seen. This complication is more prevalent in patients of rheumatoid arthritis and bronchial asthma (probably because of long duration of use), elderly subjects and post menopausal women. Alternative day therapy does not prevent this complication. Deflazacort, a synthetic oxazoline derivative of prednisone interferes with bone and mineral metabolism in a significantly lesser degree and hence may be recommended for chronic use instead of prednisolone.

Prolonged treatment with heparin in doses of 15,000 units daily causes osteoporosis with spontaneous fractures of vertebrae and ribs. This complication is prevented by lower doses (10000 U/day). The mechanisms involved include competition with chondritin sulfate to replace the normal bone matrix mucopolysaccharides, increased collagenolytic activity and potentiation of bone resorbing action of PTH. Osteoporosis is a recognized complication of drugs that reduce hypogonadism on a long term basis (e.g. GnRH analogue therapy),

Osteomalacia and Rickets

This complication is seen in about 15% of epileptics receiving long term anticonvulsant therapy. The mechanism is accelerated vitamin D catabolism by microsomal enzyme induction in the liver. Phenobarbitone and phenytoin are the most notorious while carbamazepine is relatively safe and sodium valproate has no such effects. More severe changes occur in patients receiving anticonvulsant polytherapy especially when associated with poor dietary intake of vitamin D and calcium and deficient exposure to sunlight.

Chronic laxative abuse by causing vitamin D and calcium malabsorption and aluminium containing phosphate binding antacids through hypophosphatemia may lead to osteomalacia. Bisphosphonates may cause osteomalacia by inhibiting bone turnover through their suppressive action on osteoclasts.

6. ADVERSE DRUG EFFECTS ON PITUITARY HORMONES

Hyperprolactinemia

Phenothiazines (chlorpromazine, prochlorperazine, trifluoperazine and promazine), butyrophenones (haloperidol) and prokinetic drugs (metoclopramide and domperidone) cause hyperprocatinemia by dopaminergic blockade at dopamine D2 receptors while tricyclic antidepressants, methyldopa and reserpine cause elevation in prolactin by dopamine depletion.

Histaminergic H_2 blocker cimetidine induces hyperprolactinemia while ranitidine and famotidine do so very rarely. Opiates, estrogens and benzodiazepines stimulate lactotrophs through non-dopaminergic mechanisms. These drugs cause galactorrhoea and/or amenorrhea and infertility in women and decreased libido, impotence, infertility and oligospermia in men. Phenothiazines induced galactorrhoea is estimated to occur in 10-57% of patients in various series. The effect may be dose related but duration of therapy is not important. Wide interindividual variation exists. Elevated levels of prolactin persist for 2-3 weeks after discontinuation of the drug. A thorough drugs history is important in all cases of hyperprolactinemia to obviate costly and time consuming investigations for prolactinoma.

Drugs Affecting Growth Hormone-IGF-1 Axis

Chronic glucocorticoids therapy decrease growth hormone secretion by inhibiting GHRH though in acute studies it has the opposite effect. Immunoreactive IGF-1 level are unaffected but somatomedin bioactivity is reduced and remains depressed during chronic glucocorticoids therapy. In addition, glucocorticoids have direct inhibitory action on chondrocytes in the growth plate. This adverse effect may be minimized by alternate day therapy or ACTH therapy in place of glucocorticoids, though for the latter findings are debatable. Dextroamphetamine and methylphenidate lead to growth retardation in children treated with these drugs for attention deficit hyperactivity disorders, possibly by causing anorexia, though their effects on growth hormone secretion have yet been ruled out. Androgens and anabolic steroids when used in children accelerate bone maturation and epiphyseal fusion, thereby reducing final height.

Drugs Affecting Vasopressin (ADH) Secretion and Action

Drugs like chlorpropamide, vincristine, vinblastine cyclophosphamide, carbamazepine, narcotics and tricyclic antidepressants stimulate excessive release of ADH from the neurohypophysis. Others sulfonamides (tolbutamide and glipizide) rarely have this side effect.

The consequence is SIADH (syndrome of inappropriate ADH) which occasionally leads to potential life threatening hyponatremia. The water retaining properties of antineoplastic agents are particularly important because the patient treated with these drugs is usually hydrated energetically to prevent uric acid nephropathy or cyclophosphamide induced hemorrhagic cystitis.

Nephrogenic diabetes insipidus has been observed in about 30% of patients on long-term lithium carbonate therapy. The other agents which cause this effect are demeclocycline, methoxyflurane and enflurane. The latter two anesthetic agents possibly cause this adverse effect by producing hyperoxaluria. Phenytoin has been reported to decrease ADH secretion and can precipitate diabetes insipidus in patients with underlying defects in ADH secretion.

7. ADVERSE DRUG EFFECTS ON FEMALE REPRODUCTIVE FUNCTION

Amenorrhea and Infertility

Drugs Acting through Central Mechanisms

The major drugs of this class are those which induce hyperprolactinemia as discussed already. Oral contraceptive (sequential or estrogen-progesterone combination) induced suppression of gonadotropins persists (3 months to 1 year or even more) in some women even after the 'pill' is discontinued. Possible memory effect of these drugs on GnRH-Gonadotropin axis or very rarely unmasking of an underlying prolactinoma are considered pathogenetic mechanisms. Glucocorticoids, opiates and 'the drug abuse' lead to hypogonadotropism by suppressing GnRH pulse generator.

Drugs Acting on Ovaries

Cytotoxic drugs can lend lo loss of primordial follicles with failure of both ovulation and endocrine function. Alkylating agents (e.g. cyclophosphamide) are the most gonadotoxic. The toxicity is age-dependent (less in younger patients) and progressive even after the drug is discontinued. Methotrexate is less toxic to the ovaries. Prepubertal ovaries are relatively more resistant to cytotoxic drugs probably because of low follicular activity. Normal menstrual function and fertility have been observed in women who received cyclophosphamide in childhood for the treatment of glomerulonephritis. Alkylating agents used in high doses have led to ovarian failure in many patients. Even though impaired follicular development may be reversible in some, premature menopause is a sequel. Though some reports indicate beneficial effect of suppressing ovarian activity by oral contraceptives in preventing gonadal damage, no consistent benefits has been shown. Non-steroidal antiinflammatory drugs induce ovulation by interfering with prostaglandin synthesis and thus LH effects on Graffin follicle.

Drugs Causing Virilisation

Anabolic steroids, progestogen (19-nortestosterone derivatives and danazol) cause hirsutism and other features of virilisation. Drugs like phenytoin, minoxidil, diazoxide, cyclosporine and hexachlorobenzene cause hypertrichosis without other feature of virilisation. A thorough drug history is considered important while evaluating hirsutism.

8. DRUGS AFFECTING MALE GONADAL FUNCTION

Gyanaecomastia With or Without Hypogonadism

The key factor in the pathogenesis of gynecomastia is decreased testosterone: estradiol ratio. So any drug that decreases testosterone synthesis or action or increase estrogenic activity can cause gynecomastia.

Drugs Causing Male Infertility With or Without Hypogonadism

Drugs acting directly on the testis which has predominant toxic effect on the germinal epithelium with relatively less effect on Leydig cell function induces

Table 9.2: Drug induced gynecomastia

Class/Mechanism	*Drug*
Exogenous estrogens mid estrogen	Diethyl stilboestrol, digitalis, like drugs and food containing cosmetics
Enhancers of endogens estrogens	Gonadotropins, clomiphine testosterone
Inhibitors of testosterone	Ketoconazole, metronidazole spironolactone, alkylating agents cisplatin
Inhibitors of testosterone action	Spironolactone, cimetidine cyproterone
Undefined mechanism	Busulfan, isoniazid, methyldopa, tricyclic, antidepressants, penicillamine, diazepam, marijuana, heroin

infertility. The cytotoxic drugs come under this. Alkylating drugs, procarbazine, vincristine and vinblastine are more gonadotoxic than other drugs/drug-combinations. This explains the high risk of azoospermia with MOPP and MVPP combinations used in treatment of Hodgkin's disease. Combinations containing cisplatin and bleomycin are less gonadotoxic and return of fertility has been described in patients of testicular teratoma treated with these agents. Though total loss of Leydig cell function is less common, high LH levels are found on treatment with alkylating agents, indicating compensated Leydig cell damage. Many reports have suggested that prepubertal testis is less susceptible to damage by these. Alkylating agents can damage stems cells also.

Drugs on Sperm

Sulphasalazine used for inflammatory bowel disease can produce reversible oligospermia. Drugs like cannabis also have a similar effect. Sperms mortality is also affected by chlorpromazine, imipramine, lignocaine, and beta-blockers.

CHAPTER TEN

Drug Induced Fever

Drug induced fever is a serious and confusing problem. Of medications that cause the fever the antibiotics are most frequent causes. The common antibiotic responsible for drug induces fever are beta lactams (penicillins, cephalosporins) but sulfonamides, nitrofurantoin and antituberculars can also lead to fever. Drug induced fever does not have characteristic features. Most often it occurs 5 to 10 days after the start of treatment but it may occur also right after the first dose. Most probably, the drug acts like an exogenic pyrogen. Drug fever is usually a diagnosis of exclusion. Although most patients are surprisingly well while febrile, some are profoundly septic. Fever usually subsides 48 hours after offending drug is stopped.

Many drugs can cause fever by a variety of mechanisms (Table 10.1). Drugs such as interferons can stimulate the production of endogenous pyrogens and antibacterial agents such as penicillins can kill organisms and so release endotoxins, as in the Jarisch-Herxheimer reaction. Irritant drugs can produce local phlebitis. Alterations of thermoregulation by anticholinergic agents, amphetamines including Ecstasy (methylenedioxymethamphetamine) and serotonergic agents are all important causes of drug induced fever. Antituberculous agents and anticonvulsants are implicated in fever due to hypersensitivity reactions and some drugs can cause severe hyperthermia in susceptible individuals, for example anaesthetic agents in patients predisposed to malignant hyperthermia. Drugs should be suspected in any case of fever the cause of which is obscure.

Table 10.1: Causes of drug induced fever

I. Antibiotic Induced Fever
A. Erythromycin B. Isoniazid C. Penicillin D. Nitrofurantoin E. Procainamide F. Quinidine
II. Cardiovascular Medication Induced Fever
A. Atropine B. Captopril C. Clofibrate D. Hydralazine E. Hydrochlorothiazide F. Methyldopa G. Nifedipine
III. Miscellaneous Medications Inducing Fever
A. Allopurinol B. Antihistamines C. Aspirin D. Cimetidine E. Heparin F. Meperidine G. Phenytoin

Body temperature is usually controlled within a narrow range by a number of physiological processes. It rises when heat absorption or production exceeds heat loss. Heat is absorbed from the environment and endogenous production depends on metabolic rate, muscular activity and 'non-shivering thermogenesis'. Heat is lost from the body by convection and radiation from the surface and evaporation from the skin and lungs. The normal physiological response to a rising temperature is dilatation of skin blood vessels and increased sweating.

The balance between heat production and heat loss is controlled by a combination of mechanisms including the behaviour of the whole organism (avoiding heat, shedding clothes, etc.) and homoeostatic mechanisms. Infection results in the introduction of exogenous pyrogens like bacterial lipopolysaccharide and inflammation results in the production of endogenous pyrogens, such as the cytokine interleukin-lb. These act on the preoptic region of the hypothalamus, where they lead to the production of prostaglandin E2 (PGE2) which is the neural mediator of fever, stimulating the endogenous pyrogen receptor (EP3).

A drug can cause fever in the following ways:

1. By acting as a direct or indirect pyrogen or by causing inflammation or tissue damage.
2. By causing pyrogen release as part of its pharmacological action.
3. By altering thermoregulation by central, peripheral or metabolic means.
4. By causing hypersensitivity reactions.
5. By inducing immunosuppression.
6. As a result of patient idiosyncrasy.

Drugs Acting as Direct or Indirect Pyrogens

Interferons commonly cause a "flu-like illness" with fever. They have a broad role in regulating the immune response, possibly through induction of interleukin-6, since low doses of corticosteroids reduce the symptoms at the onset of interferon beta-lb therapy in multiple sclerosis.

The immunosuppressant murumonab-CD3 (OKT3), a monoclonal antibody, causes a cytokine-release syndrome leading to fever, usually when the first dose is given. Cytokine release also seems to be the underlying mechanism in fever associated with amphotericin B infusion. Amphotericin B causes a shift towards proinflammatory cytokine production in human mononuclear cells and also stimulation of prostaglandin synthesis. Exogenous pyrogens may be administered parenterally when they contaminate a drug formulation, for example gentamicin. This is particularly seen with agents derived from microorganisms e.g. amphotericin, a mixture of antifungal polyenes produced by Streptomyces nodosus.

A local chemical phlebitis that can lead to fever, can occur with intravenous injections or infusions of antibiotics (e.g. erythromycin, vancomycin or cephalosporins), cytotoxic drugs, amiodarone, barbiturates, unemulsified diazepam and also with hypertonic fluids and solutions given for parenteral nutrition. These reactions can also become secondarily infected. Care should be taken to check all intravenous cannula sites in patients with fever. More serious local reactions such as sterile abscess formation can occur with intramuscular injections of drugs such as paraldehyde, diclofenac and gold. Drugs that cause pyrogen release by microorganisms as part of their pharmacological action.

Pyrogens Released by the Pharmacological Action of a Drug

An example of this is the Jarisch-Herxheimer reaction, in which endotoxin is released front bacteria. There is an abrupt onset of fever, myalgia, hyperventilation and tachycardia about 6-8 hours after starting bactericidal therapy with penicillin for secondary syphilis but also in other infections. The Jarisch-Hetxheimer reaction is associated with raised concentrations of tumour necrosis factor (TNF) alpha, interleukin-6 and interleukin-8. Treatment with anti-TNF-alpha Fab before giving penicillin seems to suppress the reaction.

Drugs that Interfere with Thermoregulation

Drugs can affect thermoregulation and lead to fever in several ways. Centrally, they can alter the 'set point' body temperature and alter adaptive responses to high temperature. Opioids, sedatives and alcohol can affect the ability of a person to deal with excess heat. Peripherally, drugs can reduce the ability to lose heat by vasodilatation or sweating. Metabolism can be altered leading to an increase in heat production. However, most drugs do not simply act at one level but have multiple effects, especially in overdosage. Anticholinergic agents, phenothiazines, tricyclic antidepressants, antihistamines and synthetic alkaloids impair hypothalamic function centrally and reduce sweating peripherally, leading to an anticholinergic 'toxidrome' of diminished sweating, coma, hyperreflexia, tachycardia, psychosis, dilated pupils, urinary retention, flushing and pyrexia.

The use of benztropine in combination with anti-psychotic drugs which also have anticholinergic adverse effects has been associated with fatal heat stroke when the ambient temperature is above 29°C. It may be safer to treat agitation and psychosis in anticholinergic toxicity with benzodiazepines rather than benztropine.

Profuse sweating, hyperreflexia, pyrexia, hypertonia and restlessness may be seen in toxicity with monoamine oxidase inhibitors, anticholinergic drugs, phencyclidine ('Angel dust') and amphetamine and its derivatives (such as Ecstasy).

The serotonin syndrome (Table 10.2), characterised by fever, autonomic disturbance (tachycardia), neuromuscular disorders (hyperreflexia, bizarre movements, myoclonus) and altered mental state (agitation or confusion) is caused by drugs that increase central nervous system serotonin transmission, including selective serotonin reuptake inhibitors (SSRIs). It is differentiated from the neuroleptic malignant syndrome by the drug history and by the absence of coma, Parkinsonian features or autonomic instability. In most cases, two or more types of medications known to increase the activity of serotonin at the 5HT1A receptor, or a specific interaction (an SSRI with lithium, or an SSRI with sumatriptan) or an overdose are required to produce the syndrome. As SSRIs are replacing tricyclic antidepressants, the incidence of serotonin syndrome is likely to increase. Exertional heat stroke has been reported with amphetamine analogues such as Ecstasy. Extreme physical activity induced by the stimulant effects of Ecstasy, together with high ambient temperatures and reduced water consumption, can lead to severe hyperpyrexia. Dantrolene has been used in the acute management of such cases.

Deaths from a single dose of Ecstasy may have been due to the serotonin syndrome in susceptible individuals. Epidural analgesia during labour, especially when prolonged, can cause fever in the mother and the fetus. The cause of the fever is uncertain but it may, in part, be related to the alteration of thermoregulation by the

Table 10.2: Agents causing serotonin syndrome

Antidepressants	SSRIs, monoamine oxidase inhibitors (including moclobemide), tricyclics, mirtazapine, venlafaxine
Antiparkinsonians	Amantadine, bromocriptine, levodopa, selegiline, carbergoline, pergolide
Illicit drugs	Cocaine, hallucinogenic amphetamines such as MDMA (ecstasy), LSD, etc.
Migraine therapy	Dihydroergotamine, naratriptan, sumatriptan, zolmitriptan
Other agents	Tramadol, carbamazepine, lithium, reserpine, sibutramine, St. John's wort, bupropion, pethidine, morphine

associated sympathetic blockade in epidural analgesia, which would reduce sweating.

Drugs that Cause Hypersensitivity Reactions

Hypersensitivity reactions to drugs can include fever as well as other features of hypersensitivity such as anaphylaxis (Type 1) or immune-complex disease (Type 3). Drug induced fever due to Type 3 hypersensitivity typically presents as a low-grade fever that subsequently rises. It usually starts in the first 7-10 days of drug administration, particularly with antimicrobials, although it can occur at any time. The fever subsides rapidly with drug withdrawal hut recurs within hours of rechallenge. Antimicrobials can cause fever and of course this can lead to diagnostic difficulty when there is the possibility of under treated sepsis, requiring further antimicrobial treatment. Antituberculous drugs, in particular are associated with drug fever. Rifampicin causes a 'flu-like syndrome' of fever, rigors, bone pain and malaise lasting about 12 hours after each dose when given intermittently. Other antituberculous drugs isoniazid, pyrazinamide and rarely ethambutol can also cause fever. Piperacillin has been implicated in drug fever especially in the treatment of patients with cystic fibrosis, who are often taking multiple drug regimens. Drug induced fever is seen in up to 5 per cent of patients treated with vancomycin and not uncommonly with sulphamethoxazole, trimethoprim or co-trimoxazole.

Other antibiotics implicated in drug induced fever include tetracyclines, erythromycin (in association with hepatotoxicity), imipenem, topical neomycin and nitrofurantoin. Other drugs are also particularly associated with fever. Cardiovascular drugs implicated in hypersensitivity reactions with fever include methyldopa, captopril, acetazolamide, hydralazine (in association with drug-associated lupus erythematosus), procainamide, labetalol and nifedipine. Anticonvulsants can cause fever. Carbamazepine sometimes produces a reaction with lymphadenopathy, fever, rash, hepatosplenomegaly and eosinophilia. Most cases occur within the first 30 days of starting therapy. Anticarbarnazepine antibodies have also been described. Phenobarbitone causes a fever with intensely pruritic rash. Phenytoin causes a fever with skin eruptions, lymph adenopathy and hepatitis.

Drugs that Cause Immunosuppression

Patients who are immunocompromised by cancer chemotherapy, immunosuppressants (such as azathioprine) or idiosyncratic reactions, are at risk of opportunistic infections. Cytotoxic drugs, phenothiazines, many antibiotics, NSAIDs, antithyroid agents and psychotropic drugs are among those that cause neutropenia. Fever in such patients is a common hematological emergency and management depends on rational antimicrobial use, thorough investigation and measures to reduce exposure to infection.

Idiosyncratic Drug Fever

Some individuals are especially prone to the effects of a drug and drug induced fever is one manifestation of this. Malignant hyperthermia is a dangerous hypermetabolic state after anaesthesia with suxamethonium and/or volatile halogenated anaesthetic agents. It is also seen in susceptible individuals after severe exercise in high ambient temperatures, in infections, in overheated infants and during treatment with neuroleptic drugs. It is characterised by a sustained rise in body temperature (without shivering), tachycardia, cyanosis and generalized muscle rigidity during or soon after the anaesthetic. To the non-anaesthetist, it can be mistaken for heat stroke, rhabdomyolysis, muscle pains, neuroleptic malignant syndrome or sudden infant death syndrome. Treatment consists of supportive measures, reversal of acidosis and dantrolene sodium. The genetics of malignant hyperthermia are well recognised. It is autosomal dominant but is a genetically heterogeneous condition with a variable number of genes implicated in different families. Everyone who is susceptible to malignant hyperthermia has a disorder of muscle membrane that can be demonstrated by the sensitivity of muscle biopsy strips to agents such as halothane, caffeine, potassium and temperature changes. In vitro tests can be performed to confirm susceptibility to malignant hyperthermia. Three clinical myopathies have been identified: Evans myopathy, which is usually subclinical but may have wasting of the lower thigh muscle and chronically raised creatine kinase activity; king-Denborough syndrome, which is rare and seen in young boys, small for age, with undescended testes, lordosis, kyphosis, and facial abnormalities; and central-core disease. Members of families affected by central core disease should all be assumed to be susceptible to malignant hyperthermia and there are striking microscopic changes in muscle. Neuroleptic malignant syndrome is an idiosyncratic reaction to antipsychotic drugs such as phenothiazines, butyrophenones, thioxanthenes and risperidone, but has also been seen after abrupt withdrawal of antiparkinsonian agents and treatment with dopamine-depleting agents or lithium. It is characterized by fever, hypertonia, fluctuating consciousness and autonomic disturbances such as tachycardia, sweating and labile blood pressure.

It has been argued that the syndrome may not be a rare idiosyncratic condition with a high mortality but the extreme end of a continuum of effects induced by neuroleptics, such as Parkinsonism and dystonia. Early mild cases may be far more common than previously thought. The condition is thought to be due to a profound reduction in dopaminergic function in the brain. Loss of dopamine activity in the nigrostriatal system explains the extrapyramidal effects of rigidity and Parkinsonian tremor. The sustained muscle activity then causes fever and rhabdomyolysis. Predisposing factors include physical exertion, dehydration, organic brain disease and the use of neuroleptic drugs. Lately, acquired immune deficiency syndrome (AIDS) has been suggested as another risk factor. In AIDS, there may be structural brain damage from opportunistic infections and sufferers may be more likely to suffer dehydration and to be taking many drugs. Treatment consists of withdrawal of drugs (although they may be introduced again later), supportive measures, dantrolene and dopamine receptor agonists such as bromocriptine.

Diagnosis of Drug Induced Fever

Drugs are an important, though sometimes overlooked, cause of fever and should be suspected in any case whose cause is obscure. Patients with drug induced fever tend to have been extensively investigated for bacterial infections and often treated with broad-spectrum antibiotics. In patients with fever of unknown origin, drug-related fever was the underlying cause in 5 per cent of inpatients aged over 65 years and in 3 per cent of general medical inpatients.

Drug induced fever tends to be a difficult diagnosis since it is only confirmed after the elimination of other causes, the demonstration of the link between initiation of the drug and the start of the fever and the resolution of fever within a few days of stopping the causative agent.

Any pattern of fever may be seen in drug induced fever, the mechanisms by which it occurs are numerous and many drugs have been implicated. Drugs should always be considered in the differential diagnosis of fever of obscure origin.

CHAPTER ELEVEN

Drug Induced Emergencies

Drug associated emergencies may present with a wide array of manifestations. They are common in clinical practice and are probably underreported in literature. They should enter the differential diagnosis of any new symptom or clinical deterioration in any patient on any medication. The previous chapters in this book dealt with adverse effects affecting various systems. Any of those in their more severe forms could present as an emergency.

SPECTRUM OF DRUG INDUCED EMERGENCIES

Drugs may cause emergencies in many different ways. The more common ones are discussed below:

Anaphylaxis

Anaphylaxis is probably the most dramatic of all drug induced emergencies. This is an acute and dramatic life threatening immunologic reaction to a drug. It may be mediated by IgE (anaphylactic) antibodies or by other immunogenic mechanisms (anaphylactoid). The commonest offending drugs are the beta lactam antibiotics and radiocontrast material but the reaction can be caused by a wide range of drugs. Exposure to the drug causes the release of a large number of primary mediators (from mast cells and basophiles), secondary mediators (from other inflammatory cells) and activation of various physiologic cascades. This in turn leads to widespread changes in smooth muscle tone, a leaky vasculature and tissue edema. Severe vasodilatation, bronchospasm and upper airway edema cause dyspnoea, wheeze and hypotension. Not infrequently noncardiogenic pulmonary edema may be the predominant manifestation of a drug reaction. The occurrence of this clinical picture in a few minutes of exposure to the drug is the hallmark of this reaction, though symptoms may be delayed up to six hours after exposure to the drug. A biphasic response is also known with the second reaction delayed up to six hours and being as severe as the first one. The mainstay of treatment is to limit further exposure to the drug, maintain a patent airway and administer oxygen, fluids, antihistamine agents, steroids and adrenaline

Drug Overdose

Intentional drug over dose as a method to attempt suicide (or to simulate a suicide attempt) is a common occurrence. Benzodiazepines, tricyclic antidepressants and paracetamol are among the commonly used drugs though organophosphorus compounds are probably the most frequently used agents for this purpose. The clinical presentation will depend on the quantity of drug taken.

Benzodiazepines overdose presents with coma and respiratory depression, tricyclic agents with the same presentation but with additional dysrrhythmias and paracetamol with a delayed but fulminant hepatic failure. Unintentional drug overdose may occur due to faulty prescribing, failing to prescribe tablet strength on prescriptions or in patients in whom drug elimination is decreased due to hepatic or renal dysfunction and the dose is not decreased appropriately.

Increased Sensitivity to Drugs

Some patients may be sensitive to drugs which can potentially cause respiratory or circulatory depression. This is commonly seen in elderly patients and those who are sick or critically ill in whom normal doses of drugs can cause hypotension or respiratory depression. Hypovolemic patients may have a severe fall of blood pressure with normal doses of drugs that cause cardiac depression or vasodilatation.

Erroneous Prescription

Failure to prescribe a drug legibly occasionally leads to tragic emergencies. The author is aware of cases where pancuronium, a paralyzing anesthetic agent was administered instead of pethidine with a fatal outcome, digoxin given instead of dulcolax resulted in severe vomiting and arrhythmias and adrenaline given instead of atropine caused ventricular tachyarrhythmia, methotrexate given daily instead of weekly leading to fatal bone marrow depression. Another source of drug associated emergency occurs when one patient receives another patient's prescription. This is more likely occur when patients with common surnames (e.g. Singh, Shah, Mehta) are in the same ward. Careful attention to detail is the only way to prevent such emergencies. All prescriptions should be in capital letters, doctor and nurse drug charts should be frequently cross checked. The practice of two nurses checking and countersigning each drug administration is mandatory in some countries and should be introduced and encouraged in our country.

Inappropriate Use of Drugs

The use of beta blockers in patients with asthma, COPD or cardiac failure may precipitate an episode of respiratory failure or pulmonary edema. Similarly sedatives used in patient with hepatic disease may result in encephalopathy and when use in those with COPD may cause severe hypoventilation or even respiratory arrest.

Direct Side Effect of A Drug

Almost all drugs have side effects and some of these will present as emergencies. NSAIDs may cause hypovolemic shock due to massive blood loss, anti-diabetic agents may cause hypoglycemic coma, and anticoagulants may cause an intracerebral haemorrhage. Almost any adverse reaction to a drug described in this book could lead to an emergency.

Indirect Side Effects

Occasionally the presentation of an emergency may not be directly due to the side effect of the drug but due to a secondary effect. Aminoglycosides induced renal failure may present as fulminant pulmonary edema or with a hyperkalemia crisis. Similarly severe sepsis may be the presenting manifestation of a drug induces neutropenia or immune suppression.

Anaesthetic Drugs

All anesthetic drugs are potent agents capable of severely compromising the airway, breathing and circulation. As anesthesia is given in controlled circumstances these are usually appropriately supported. However a light hearted approach to anaesthetic agents, their use by comparatively inexperienced doctors, inadequate monitoring during anaesthesia often results in cardio-respiratory compromise and occasionally to cardio-respiratory arrest in otherwise completely healthy patients. Administering anaesthesia to sick patients or to patients with chronic cardiorespiratory disease may have significant complications. Additionally anaphylactic reactions of prolonged paralysis may result from exposure to anaesthetic agents in susceptible patients.

Blood and Blood Products

Good blood banking practices have now rendered blood transfusion safe. Mismatched transfusion however still, rarely occurs and presents with rigor, circulatory collapse and acute renal failure. Massive transfusion can result in coagulopathy and the adult respiratory distress syndrome (ARDS).

Oxygen Toxicity

The excess use of oxygen in patients with COPD and chronic hypercarbia may precipitate an episode of ventilatory failure. However it must be stressed that hypoxemia is more dangerous than hypoventilation and the practice of depriving the severely hypoxemic patient of oxygen to prevent hypoventilation must be strongly discouraged.

Hypotension

In patients presenting with hypotension as a drug induced emergency rapid fluid infusion should be started after ensuring that the patient is not in pulmonary edema or cardiac failure. Most drug induced hypotension is due to a combination of venodilation with resultant decrease in venous return and an additional arterial vasodilation with a subsequent fall in the systemic vascular resistance. The use of inotropic agents like dopamine is inappropriate as a first line of therapy as the primary problem is a peripheral pooling of blood. Infusion of 0.5-1 liter of fluid usually corrects most drug associated hypotension. In anaphylaxis however there is extreme vasodilation and a leaky vasculature and the amount of fluid required to adequately fill the circulation may be as high a 6-9 liters.

Only when adequate fluid replacement does not stabilize the circulation should inotropic therapy be considered. An indwelling arterial catheter should be inserted to allow continuous monitoring of the blood pressure. A central venous catheter should be inserted prior to starting the inotrope infusion. This catheter is necessary for both CVP monitoring and inotrope infusion.

If feasible a triple lumen catheter should be used with one lumen used only for inotrope administration. This will prevent swings of blood pressure due to sudden increases or decreases of inotrope being delivered when the same lumen is used for CVP monitoring or other drug bolus administration. Rarely a patient with drug overdose may have refractory hypotension due to severe arterial vasodilation. A pulmonary artery catheter is necessary to guide therapy.

Typical findings in such a situation include high central venous and pulmonary artery wedge pressures, a very high cardiac index of 1.5-2 times of normal and a very low systemic vascular resistance of (less than 33% of normal). In this clinical setting the careful use of noradrenalin as a vasopressin infusion will correct the hypotension. This therapy should be guided with a pulmonary artery catheter as excess vasoconstriction will reverse the hypotension but may decrease organ perfusion. Hourly urine output measurement is a simple way of assessing organ perfusion and should be used in all patients with an unstable circulation.

SPECIFIC DIAGNOSIS AND THERAPY

As soon as the physiological status of the patient is stable, focus of management should shift to establishing a complete diagnosis and instituting specific therapy. It must be stressed again that this usually proceeds simultaneously with physiological evaluation and support in all but the most unstable patients. A complete history, review of drug charts (both doctors and nurses charts), and a review of any old notes will help identify the offending drug and any chronic illness which have caused the present emergency.

Specific treatment will depend completely on the nature of the illness. As mentioned previously, further doses of the offending drug should be withheld. If the emergency is due to overdose, the antidote, if available, should be administered. Further absorption should be limited with a stomach wash and nasogastric activated charcoal administration. Elimination too can occasionally be enhanced with a forced acid or alkaline diuresis. If the drug has induced a specific, problem this should be treated appropriately. Beta blocker induced bronchospasm can be reversed with bronchodilators, NSAID induced stomach bleeds can be treated with adequate blood replacement and antiulcer agents and anticoagulant induced intracranial bleed corrected with vitamin K and FFP with additional surgical evacuation if necessary. Similarly if the problem is a neutropenia induced sepsis, antibiotics should be administered and those presenting with fluid over load should be treated with diuretics and haemofilteration or dialysis if necessary. Technical problems resulting in an emergency e.g. rapid or blocked infusion are easily corrected if rapidly identified.

Drug induced emergencies are common in clinical practice and may be life threatening. They may pre sent in many varied ways and should be considered in the differential diagnosis of any emergency in any patient on, any medication. Management consists of correcting the primary drug associated emergency and supporting the cardiopulmonary systems till the problem has been adequately dealt with and the drug eliminated from the body.

CHAPTER TWELVE

ADRs Associated with Drug Interactions

Drug interactions deserve a special mention because interactions are one of the leading causes of the ADRs. Drug interactions are often recognized only when toxicity occurs. Sufficient knowledge regarding effective and safe use of drugs is possible only if there is adequate understanding of pharmacokinetic and pharmacodynamic of drugs, thus enabling physicians to select proper drug combinations. Estimates of the numbers of patients injured due to drug interactions vary widely. In a systems analysis of ADRs, it was estimated that drug-drug interactions represent from 3-5% of all in hospital medication errors. Drug interactions are also an important cause of patient visits to emergency departments.

It has been estimated that drug interactions may be fourth to sixth leading cause of death in hospitalised patients in United States. Drug interactions between drugs represent a major concern for the pharmaceutical industry, for regulatory agencies and clinically for health care professionals and their patients. Drug interactions may be synergistic or antagonistic, desired or undesired, beneficial or harmful. Most drug interactions would be of Type A. Clinical case reports or studies usually provide the first evidence of interaction between drugs.

DRUG INTERACTION CAN OCCUR AT 3 LEVELS (Table 12.1)

1. PHARMACEUTICAL

These are interactions before administration. These interactions can occur in vitro (I.V. fluid, syringe, vial) due to chemical interaction, e.g., heparin should not be mixed with tetracyclines, penicillins and hydrocortisone in the same syringe. Inactivation of these drugs may occur.

When phenytoin is added to solutions of dextrose, a precipitate forms and the phenytoin falls to the bottom of the i.v. bag as an insoluble salt. When this happens, it is no longer available to control seizures. Amphotericin is still used widely as a urinary bladder perfusion to treat aggressive fungal infections. If it is administered in saline, the drug precipitates and can erode through the bladder wall if not removed. The clinical presentation of such cases is an acute abdomen due to perforation of the bladder. Lastly, it is recommended that aminoglycosides not be co-mixed in I.V. fluids with betalactam antibiotics. This can markedly reduce antibiotic efficacy.

Table 12.1: Sites of adverse drug interaction

Site	*Mechanism*
In vitro	I.V. route
Oral	Bioavailability
Intestine	Altered absorption
Liver	Enzyme induction/inhibition
Plasma	Protein binding
Kidney	Reabsorption, secretion pH, pKa effect
Receptor	Competition /antagonism

2. PHARMACOKINETIC

More often the cause of drug interaction is an alteration of pharmacokinetic processes of one drug by another. Pharmacokinetic process can be altered during absorption, distribution, metabolism or excretion of drugs.

Absorption

Drug interactions can take place during absorption of drugs in the GI Tract. Particularly notable among these is the ability of aluminum-containing medicines such as sucralfate and antacids to reduce the absorption of expensive and potentially life-saving antibiotics like ciprofloxacin and azithromycin. Women taking iron supplements often do not consider them as medicines and should be specifically questioned about whether they are taking iron if they are to be prescribed a quinolone or azithromycin. Drugs such as ketoconazole and delavirdine require an acidic environment to be in the non-charged form that is preferentially absorbed. Solubility is drastically reduced in neutral or basic medications such as omeprazole, lansoprazole or H_2-antagonists that raise the stomach's pH.

The following drugs/food products i.e.:

- Sucralfate, some milk products, antacids, and oral iron preparations.
- Omeprazole, lansoprazole, H_2-antagonists.
- Didanosine (given as a buffered tablet).
- Cholestyramine.
- Block absorption of quinolones, tetracycline, and azithromycin.
- Reduce absorption of ketoconazole, delavirdine.
- Reduces ketoconazole absorption.
- Binds raloxifene, thyroid hormone, and digoxin.

Distribution

Displacement of highly protein bound drug (oral anticoagulant) by another drug (e.g. NSAIDs) could lead to an increase in the free concentration of first drug and an adverse effect (bleeding tendency). But most of the drug interactions due to plasma protein displacement reactions are not clinically significant, because the displaced drug is eliminated faster i.e. more free drug is now available to kidneys for elimination.

Metabolism

Drug interactions involving metabolism are clinically the most important drug interactions. Some important preventable drug interactions are due to their effects on drug metabolizing enzymes, resulting in either inhibition (reduced activity) of the enzyme or induction (increased activity) of the enzyme. There are many potential consequences of changes in drug metabolism for a given drug. It is made more complex by the fact that there are multiple pathways of metabolism for many drugs.

The major group of enzymes in the liver that metabolize drugs can be isolated in a subcellular fraction termed the microsomes. The largest and most important of these enzymes are the cytochrome P_{450} (CYP_{450}) family of enzymes. In addition to CYP_{450}, there are other enzymes in microsomes such as flavin monooxygenase (termed FMO3). These are also responsible for metabolism of some drugs, but have not been as well characterized as the cytochrome P_{450} system. There are some characteristics of drug metabolism that can help predict important interactions due to inhibition of metabolism. Since Phase II reactions generally result in conjugation of a drug to a water-soluble group like a sugar, peptide (glutathione) or sulfur group and because there is a large excess of these groups in well nourished cells, these reactions are rarely rate-limiting. Thus, they are rarely involved in drug interactions. In contrast, the Phase I reactions carried out by cytochrome P_{450} enzymes, flavin monooxygenases and reductases are more frequently rate limiting. These are the target of clinically significant drug interactions, such as the inhibition of cyclosporine metabolism by erythromycin.

Several recent studies discuss such drug interactions at the molecular or enzyme level and therefore constitute an important link between clinical and experimental research. Central to this approach is an understanding of the catalytic importance of individual CYP_{450} isoenzymes in particular metabolic pathways. The CYP_{450} enzyme family plays a dominant role in the biotransformation of a vast number of structurally diverse drugs. The cytochrome P_{450} system performs this function by oxidising, hydrolysing or reducing the chemicals. This enables another group of enzymes, conjugation enzymes, to attach polar groups to make the metabolites water soluble so that they can be excreted in the urine. Although there are other enzyme systems that perform similar functions, the cytochrome P_{450} system is important because it is involved in most clinically relevant metabolic drug interactions. Six CYP_{450} isoforms are clinically important.

Factors Affecting Activity of Cytochrome P_{450}

There are several factors that influence CYP_{450} activity directly or at enzyme regulation level.

Enzyme Inhibition/Induction

Many drug interactions are a result of inhibition or induction of CYP_{450} enzymes. Inhibition based drug interactions form a major part of clinically significant drug interactions. Six isoenzymes of the CYP enzyme system CYP3A4, CYP2D6, CYP1A2, CYP2C9, CYP2C19 and CYP2E1 are mainly involved in metabolism of the most of the drugs. CYP3A4 isoenzyme is the most predominant isoenzyme in the liver and is involved in the metabolism of approximately 30-40% of drugs. CYP2D6 accounts for less than 2% of the total content of P_{450} in the liver, but is responsible for the metabolism of a large fraction of drugs.

The majority of drugs that are metabolized are converted to inactive metabolites. This is the most common fate for most drugs. Of the remaining drugs, some are converted to metabolites that retain the same activity as the parent. An example of this is fexofenadine, the active metabolite of terfenadine that has equal potency at the histamine receptor and now is on the market and used clinically for allergic rhinitis. However, fexofenadine is more than 50 times less active in blocking potassium channels in the heart and therefore, unlike terfenadine, does not cause torsades de pointes. In some cases the metabolites are actually more potent than the parent. For example, a prodrug such as enalapril must be hydrolyzed to enalaprilat to become active. In some cases, the metabolites have entirely new pharmacologic actions not seen with the parent drug. Metabolites can also be toxic, such as the metabolites of acetaminophen, which can cause liver failure or the metabolite of meperidine, which can cause seizures.

Inhibition of metabolism could result in potentially toxic concentrations of the parent compound. On the other hand, if the parent drug needs to be metabolized to the active compound and metabolism is inhibited, then a therapeutic failure could result. This happens, for example, if codeine a prodrug is not metabolized to morphine. Induction of drug metabolizing enzymes could similarly result in a subtherapeutic effect by reducing drug levels below that required for efficacy. Also note that CYP3A is found in the liver and also in the GI tract. Drugs that are substrates of CYP3A can be extensively metabolized in the GI tract. Infact, the GI tract is responsible for a large part of the metabolism that was formerly attributed totally to the liver. Inhibition of GI tract CYP3A also results in higher plasma levels of substrate drugs.

Clinically significant interactions occur when one drug affects the metabolism of another causing a change in concentration. This change in concentration can have clinical implications depending on the concentration-effect relationship. A number of factors influence this, including:

- The position of the drug concentration on the dose-response curve at the time of the interaction.
- The slope of the concentration-effect curve.
- The size of the change in concentration of the drug.
- The therapeutic index of the drug.

If the drug concentration is near the top of the response curve, adding a drug that increases its concentration will not increase its efficacy, regardless of the size of the interaction. However, the increase in concentration still may be relevant with respect to toxicity. An example of this is with drugs that increase the concentration of amlodipine. Increasing the concentration beyond a certain point does not increase the hypotensive effect.

As a general rule, if an enzyme inhibitor doubles the concentration, an enhanced drug response/toxicity can occur. However, even a small increase may be toxic for medications with a narrow therapeutic index. Likewise a small decrease may be important for medications (such as cyclosporin) that rely on a certain concentration for their efficacy. Drugs which induce or inhibit the enzymes of cytochrome P_{450} should ring alarm bells. Interacting drugs with a low therapeutic index are likely to be affected by even small changes in concentration.

Patient Factors

Gender, hormonal status, age and pre-existing conditions can all affect whether a drug interaction is likely to be clinically significant. For example, giving high doses of cisapride to someone with a normal heart or normal doses to someone with a long QT interval, will increase the likelihood of an arrhythmia. Drugs which reduce cisapride metabolism by inhibiting CYP3A4 (e.g. macrolides) can increase its concentration and further increase the chance of a potentially fatal arrhythmia occurring.

Genetic Polymorphism

Some people have mutations in one or more of the nucleic acids in the DNA sequence expressing a given cytochrome P_{450} isozyme. As a result, the enzyme may be absent or have low or no metabolizing activity for drugs that are usually metabolized by that enzyme. If the mutation is relatively common (more than 1%) it creates a polymorphism. This is a trait that has genetic variation that results in more than a single population being represented in greater than 1% of the total population. It literally means that the distribution of the trait has "multiple", "forms", i.e. "poly", "morphic". At least 3 of the cytochrome P_{450}s (2D6, 2C19, 2C9) are polymorphic in their distribution. People expressing a polymorphism will therefore metabolize drugs at a different rate than the rest of the population.

There is tremendous variability between individuals in terms of expression of cytochrome P_{450} isozymes. For example, CYP2D6 is not present at all in some livers. Genetic polymorphism leads to expressing high or low activities of certain enzymes. A population may be poor or fast metaboliser for a particular drug. About 5-10% of Caucasians and 1% of Asians are poor metaboliser of drugs metabolised by CYP$%) isoenzyme 2D69. Poor metabolisers are more prone to adverse drug reactions because metabolism is decreased and blood levels are high. Polymorphism of 2D6 contributes to the pronounced interindividual variability observed in the elimination of important drugs including tricyclic antidepressants, antipsychotics, mexiletine and several b-adrenergic receptor blockers. About 5% of whites and 20% of Asians are poor metaboliser of drugs metabolised by isoenzyme 2C19. The frequency of poor metabolisers in Indian population is about 11-20%. The Chinese are poor metabolisers of 2C19 and are more prone to sedative effect of diazepam and they are prescribed lower doses of diazepam.

Administration

The route of administration and the timing of a dose can be important. Oral administration is more likely to have cytochrome P_{450} interactions because the drug is then subject to cytochrome P_{450} interactions in the gut wall as well as in the liver. An example of this is grapefruit juice. When taken at the same time as felodipine, it inhibits gut wall CYP3A4, increasing felodipine absorption across the gut wall and therefore bioavailability.

First-Pass Metabolism

In general, if a drug has a high first-pass metabolism through the liver one can expect a marked increase in its concentration if it is taken with another drug which inhibits metabolism. This may lead to increased toxicity. Examples of drugs which undergo first-pass metabolism by CYP3A4 include:

- Very high first-pass metabolism: buspirone, ergotamine, lovastatin, nimodipine, saquinavir, simvastatin.
- High first-pass metabolism: oestradiol, atorvastatin, felodipine, indinavir, isradipine, nicardipine, propafenone and tacrolimus.

- Intermediate first-pass metabolism: amiodarone, carbamazepine, carvedilol, cisapride, cyclosporin, diltiazem, ethinyloestradiol, etoposide, losartan, midazolam, nifedipine, nelfinavir, ondansetron, pimozide, sildenafil, triazolam and verapamil.

Significant Interactions by Drug Class

Anticonvulsants

Carbamazepine, oxcarbamazepine, and phenytoin reduce the concentration of oral contraceptives by inducing CYP3A4. This has resulted in some women having unplanned pregnancies. Carbamazepine toxicity has occurred with 3A4 inhibitors. Phenytoin reduces the concentrations of many drugs metabolised by the cytochrome P_{450} system. This results in clinically significant effects for some drugs with a low therapeutic index such as warfarin and cyclosporin.

Immunosuppressants

Ketoconazole widely inhibits the cytochrome P_{450} system and doubles the oral availability of concurrently administered cyclosporin. This interaction has been used to enable patients to be given lower doses of cyclosporin. Other inhibitors of CYP3A4 have been used with similar, but less predictable results. Tacrolimus is a substrate for CYP3A4. Clinically significant toxicity has been reported when co-administered with CYP3A4 inhibitors, such as diltiazem. CYP3A4 inducers such as carbamazepine reduce tacrolimus concentrations. St John's wort has caused organ rejection when added to cyclosporin therapy, by inducing CYP3A4.

Protease Inhibitors

Ritonavir, a CYP3A4 inhibitor, is often added to saquinavir, a CYP3A4 substrate, as their interaction results in a 33% increase in the maximum concentration of saquinavir. Grapefruit juice can double the bioavailability of saquinavir, although this is not reliable enough to be used clinically. St John's wort, a CYP3A4 inducer, reduces the concentration of indinavir, a CYP3A4 substrate, by 57%. This is clinically significant as the reduction can lead to failure of therapy.

Anti-infectives

Ketoconazole and to a lesser extent itraconazole inhibit all cytochrome P_{450} enzymes. These antifungal drugs can cause many clinically significant interactions by increasing the concentrations of other drugs. Fluconazole has clinically significant interactions only if the other drug has a low therapeutic index, e.g. cyclosporin. Miconazole oral gel increases the INR in patients taking warfarin, hence increases chances of bleeding. Erythromycin has similar interactions with ketoconazole. Rifampicin is an enzyme inducer and has been reported to reduce the concentration of drugs metabolised by cytochrome P_{450}.

Cardiovascular

Felodipine concentrations are increased by grapefruit juice, erythromycin and itraconazole, but the change in blood pressure is not usually significant. It is more likely to be a problem in people who cannot tolerate even a small reduction in blood pressure. Diltiazem and verapamil increase the concentration of cyclosporin and, because of cyclosporin's low therapeutic index, this is likely to be clinically significant.

Pimozide can cause QT prolongation by themselves if their concentrations are high enough. However, this effect will occur more frequently if the drugs are taken with CYP3A4 inhibitors such as diltiazem, macrolides, ketoconazole or grapefruit juice.

Rhabdomyolysis occurs more frequently with increasing concentration of 'statins'. The risk may be increased when statins such as the predominantly CYP3A4 metabolised lovastatin, simvastatin and atorvastatin are given with CYP3A4 inhibitors like macrolides, diltiazem and grapefruit juice.

Warfarin has a complex metabolic pathway acting as a substrate for a number of cytochrome P_{450} enzymes.

Any change in medication in patients on warfarin requires close monitoring of the INR for a period long enough to ensure the plasma concentrations are at steady state. For example, when amiodarone, which has a half-life of 26-107 days, is added to or subtracted from warfarin it may not have its full impact on the INR for 100-400 days.

Antidepressants

Some selective serotonin reuptake inhibitors (SSRIs) (e.g. fluoxetine, paroxetine and fluvoxamine) inhibit CYP2D6. If a patient taking one of these drugs is given codeine, it cannot be converted to morphine. This results in lack of analgesic activity. The same drugs have been reported to prolong the INR when used with warfarin. Paroxetine has also caused a serious interaction by inhibiting the metabolism of perhexilene.

Nefazodone is a substrate and an inhibitor of CYP3A4. It increases the concentration of several CYP3A4 substrates including cisapride, terfenadine, astemizole and pimozide. This may cause arrhythmias. Similarly nefazodone reduces the required doses of triazolam and alprazolam by 75% and 50% respectively. Death from rhabdomyolysis has been reported, due to the addition of nefazodone to simvastatin, a CYP3A4 substrate.

Tricyclic antidepressants and SSRIs should not routinely be used together as the combination can result in a serotonergic syndrome. Most tricyclics are extensively metabolised by CYP2D6 and concentrations will increase if an inhibitory drug e.g. an SSRI is co-administered. The addition of fluoxetine, paroxetine or fluvoxamine (CYP2D6 inhibitors) to patients on desipramine, imipramine or nortriptyline results in a clinically significant (but often unpredictable) increase in tricyclic concentration.

Others

The concentration of oral contraceptives may be reduced by enzyme inducers. This interaction is clinically relevant with griseofulvin, rifampicin and carbamazepine. Sildenafil is a substrate of CYP3A4. It should not be prescribed with CYP3A4 inhibitors as they increase its concentration and therefore the likelihood of systemic hypotensive effects.

Individual Isoenzymes

Table 12.2 shows individual isoenzymes, their inhibitors and inducers.

CYP3A

CYP3A is the drug metabolizing pathway involved in the case of torsades de pointes described earlier. Terfenadine, one of the first non-sedating antihistamines, is metabolized by CYP3A to fexofenadine. When the CYP3A-mediated metabolism of terfenadine is inhibited by ketoconazole, as in the case described, terfenadine accumulates to high levels. At these high levels, terfenadine is a blocker of potassium channels in the heart. Potassium channels are important for repolarization of the heart. Once these channels are blocked, QT interval on the electrocardiogram can be prolonged and torsades de pointes can develop, as was seen in this case. Many commonly used drugs can inhibit this enzyme. This important enzyme has been the basis for most of the fatal drug interactions that have gained so much publicity in recent years. For terfenadine, as well as astemizole and cisapride, recognition and reporting of torsades de pointes in association with these drug and its interactions ultimately led to withdrawal of these drugs from the market.

These are the important inhibitors of CYP3A that will make patients appear phenotypically to resemble poor metabolizers. Azole antifungal drugs, in general, are potent inhibitors of CYP3A, although fluconazole is a weak inhibitor and inhibits CYP3A only at high doses. All the macrolide antibiotics, except azithromycin, are also potent inhibitors of this cytochrome P_{450} isoform. Cimetidine is a broad, but relatively weak, inhibitor of many cytochrome P_{450} enzymes. Also, notice that a food, grapefruit juice, is listed as an inhibitor. Several commonly used drugs have been characterized as inducers of CYP3A. Use of these drugs could potentially result in lack of therapeutic efficacy of a CYP3A substrate.

Table 12.2: Cytochrome P_{450} isoenzymes, their substrates, inhibitors and inducers

Iso-enzyme	Substrates	Inhibitors	Inducers
3A	Most calcium channel blockers Most benzodiaze-pines Most HIV protease inhibitors Most statins Cyclosporine Most non-sedating antihistamines	Ketoconazole Fluconazole Cimetidine Erythromycin Troleandomycin Grapefruit juice	Carbama-zepine Rifampin Rifabutin Ritonavir St. John's wort
2D6	Codeine Many tricyclic antidepressants	SSRIs Haloperidol Amiodarone Metoclopramide	Dexa methasone Rifampicin
2C9	Most NSAIDs (including COX-2) S-warfarin (the active form) Phenytoin	Fluconazole Fluvastatin Isoniazid Sulfamethoxazole Zafirlukast	Rifampicin Secobarbital
2C19	Diazepam Phenytoin Omeprazole	Omeprazole Isoniazid Ketoconazole	Carbamaze-pine pentob-arbital Rifampicin
1A2	Theophylline Imipramine Propranolol Clozapine	Many fluoro-quinolone antibiotics Fluvoxamine Cimetidine	Brussel sprouts Char-grilled meat Omeprazole Tobacco

CYP2D6

CYP2D6 metabolizes many of the cardiovascular and neurologic drugs in use today. Study of CYP2D6 has led to understanding the failure of codeine to relieve pain in some patients. Codeine is actually a prodrug that is converted to morphine. Codeine itself is much less active as an analgesic, but causes nausea and other adverse effects. The absence of cytochrome P_{450} 2D6 in 7% of Caucasians means that these individuals cannot metabolize codeine to the active metabolite, morphine, and therefore will get little, if any, pain relief from codeine. However, they will experience codeine's adverse effects, particularly if the dose is increased in the futile attempt to obtain pain relief.

Thirty percent of Ethiopians studied had multiple copies of the 2D6 gene (up to 13) and increased enzyme activity resulting in ultrarapid metabolism. Ultra-rapid metabolism results in lower blood levels following a standard dose of any drug metabolized by this enzyme. Therefore these patients may have an inadequate response to standard dosages of ß-blockers, narcotic analgesics or antidepressants and may require higher dosages for clinical effectiveness.

Several commonly used medications inhibit CYP2D6. These include quinidine as well as haloperidol and some other antipsychotics. The well-described pharmacokinetic interaction between selective serotonin reputake inhibitor (SSRI) antidepressants and tricyclic antidepressants appears to be due to the fact that fluoxetine and paroxetine are both potent inhibitors of CYP2D6 and render patients metabolically equivalent to people who do not have the enzyme. This increases the plasma levels of tricyclic antidepressants and increases the potential for side effects. In contrast, patients co-prescribed fluoxetine or paroxetine with codeine may experience no analgesic benefit.

CYP2C9

CYP2C9 has a polymorphic distribution in the population and is missing in 1% of Caucasians. It is the major enzyme responsible for metabolism of many of the non-steroidal anti-inflammatory drugs (NSAIDs), including the second generation cyclooxygenase-2 (COX-2) specific inhibitors. A number of other important medications have their metabolism primarily catalyzed by CYP2C9. An important drug metabolized by this enzyme is warfarin, and almost all inter-patient variability in warfarin levels and anticoagulant effects can be explained on the basis of CYP2C9 activity (not the differences in protein binding as originally thought).

The azole antifungal agent fluconazole is a potent inhibitor of CYP2C9. Fluconazole, at conventional doses, abolishes CYP2C9 activity. An interaction between fluconazole and warfarin results in at least a two-fold increase in warfarin blood level, a reduction in warfarin clearance and increased anticoagulation. Clinical studies have identified a significant interaction between fluconazole and celecoxib, leading to a twofold increase in celecoxib plasma concentrations. A clinical pharmacokinetic study demonstrated an increase in phenytoin area under the plasma concentration curve (AUC) following fluconazole administration and symptomatic phenytoin toxicity has been reported with concomitant administration of fluconazole and phenytoin.

CYP2C19

Cytochrome P_{450} 2C19 is notable because of its genetic absence in such a high percentage of Asians (approximately 20–30%). This enzyme metabolizes many anticonvulsants, diazepam, omeprazole and several of the tricyclic antidepressants. Asians have reduced clearance of diazepam compared to Caucasians and in fact, a survey of Asian and Western physicians demonstrated the use of lower doses of diazepam in Asians. Asian patients may have a lower omeprazole dosage requirement for effective treatment of *Helicobacter pylori*. According to the omeprazole package insert, Asians have about a four-fold increase in the AUC of omeprazole compared to Caucasians and the labelling recommends that one should consider dosage adjustment. In addition, the poor metabolizer genotype for CYP2C19 resulted in a higher cure rate for *H. pylori* (100%) than the rapid metabolizer genotype (28.6%) in an Asian population treated with omeprazole as part of dual therapy. Similar results have been shown more recently with proton pump inhibitors in a triple therapy regimen.

Ketoconazole and omeprazole are inhibitors of CYP2C19 and have the potential for clinically significant interactions with substrates of CYP2C19 such as diazepam or phenytoin. Isoniazid, used to treat tuberculosis, is an inhibitor of CYP2C19 and should be prescribed cautiously to patients taking phenytoin and other drugs metabolized by CYP2C19.

CYP1A2

Cytochrome P_{450} 1A2 is an important drug metabolizing enzyme in the liver that metabolizes many commonly used drugs including theophylline, imipramine, propranolol and clozapine. CYP1A2 is induced in a clinically relevant manner by tobacco smoking. The clearance of theophylline, imipramine, propranolol and clozapine are all increased by smoking. Thus, people who smoke may require higher doses of some of the medications that are substrates of CYP1A2. In contrast, a smoker would require a decrease in theophylline dosage if, for example, smoking were discontinued and the enzyme no longer induced.

Inhibitors of CYP1A2, including some fluoroquinolone antibiotics, can increase the plasma concentrations of drugs that are metabolized by CYP1A2 with a potential for increased toxicity.

Our knowledge of the isoenzymes involved in metabolism of drugs will allow a prediction of interactions of these drugs with new drugs, to be developed in the future. Indeed an editorial from US FDA suggests that this type of information will be required for future new drugs.

The cytochrome P_{450} enzymes have 3 interesting properties that often make it possible to predict drug interactions.

First, genetic polymorphism as discussed above.

Second, people that have usual drug metabolizing ability can become phenotypic poor metabolizers if they are given a substance (drug or food as we will see later) that inhibits the enzyme. So if two drugs are given that are metabolized by the same enzyme and one inhibits the enzyme, the second drug can accumulate to higher and potentially toxic levels.

Third, several of the cytochrome P_{450} isozymes can be "induced" to have increased activity. If this occurs, metabolism of any drug that is a substrate for that isozyme will be metabolized more quickly resulting in lower plasma concentrations of the drug. This may also reduce the efficacy of the drug. Also, if the drug is metabolized to a toxic compound, the toxic metabolite may accumulate to higher levels.

Table 12.3: Drugs removed from or restricted in the U.S. market because of drug interactions

1. Terfenadine February 1998
2. Mibefradil) June 1998
3. Astemizole July 1999
4. Cisapride January 2000

Mibefradil, terfenadine and cisapride provide classical examples indicating the critical importance of CYP enzyme mediated drug interactions in the development, regulation and ultimate economic success of drugs. The inability of the FDA to effectively warn health care providers and patients about drug interactions and our inability to translate existing knowledge into changes in prescribing have resulted in huge economic consequences for the pharmaceutical industry and the loss from the marketplace of effective drugs, including terfenadine, mibefradil, astemizole and cisapride.

These 4 drugs were removed from the market or restricted in their use because it became clear that they continued to be prescribed in an unsafe manner, even after multiple warning letters were disseminated by the manufacturer and the FDA to health care professionals concerning their proper use. Each of these drugs has value in the pharmaceutical marketplace and each has value to patients. However, because the manufacturer and the FDA could not prevent co-prescription of these drugs with interacting drugs resulting in fatal interactions, the risk associated with continued widespread availability could not be justified.

Excretion

Drugs can compete for excretion, hence inhibiting excretion. This leads to increased concentration and hence toxicity e.g. sulfinpyrazone inhibits excretion of tolbutamide.

3. PHARMACODYNAMIC

Pharmacodynamic interaction occurs at site of action. The combined inhibitory effects of propranolol and verapamil or diltiazem on atrioventricular node represent potential site of an adverse interaction. Alteration of compensatory mechanisms could also lead to such interactions. Beta blockers prolong the recovery from hypoglycemic effects of antidiabetics. Finally, interactions can occur at the level of drug action, such as the combination of verapamil, a calcium channel blocker and a beta-blocker. Both slow the heart rate by different mechanisms and the combination is relatively contraindicated because heart block can result. Because of this interaction many textbooks and computer programs warn against concomitant use of any beta-blocker and any calcium channel blocker. This creates a great deal of confusion and distrust of drug interaction warnings, because most health care providers know that drugs in these two classes are often employed successfully and safely in patients with hypertension.

Effects of Drug Interactions

1. Diminished therapeutic response.
2. Enhanced side effects.
3. Relative overdosage toxicity.
4. Intensified allergic reactions.
5. Increased secondary effects.
6. Severe idiosyncratic reactions.
7. Greater teratogenicity.
8. Additive addiction potential.
9. Miscellaneous.

Diminished Therapeutic Response (Also Considered Adverse Event)

Diminished therapeutic response is likely to be more often detected if the clinician monitors the magnitude of therapeutic response according to preset quantitative criteria. A reduction in therapeutic response could be due to:

1. A decreased plasma level of the drug, which in turn may be due to a diminished absorption, an increased protein-binding, an enhanced metabolism or a rapid excretion of the active drug.
2. A reduced response of the target tissue either due to a passive occupation of the receptors by the other drug or an opposite pharmacodynamic effect of the other drug.

There are many examples of drug interaction causing diminished therapeutic response. The binding of tetracyclines by antacids or calcium salts has been cited very often. However, in India, we must also consider the possibilities of decreased absorption of tetracyclines when a patient may be concurrently consuming an Ayurvedic drug e.g. Kapardikn-Bhasma (Calcined seashells) containing calcium. Methyl-dopa and Levodopa may compete for the same enzyme and if given together may diminish their respective therapeutic response. Drugs stimulating the drug metabolism can decrease the plasma level of other drug and hence diminish therapeutic response.

Enhanced Side Effects

When the drugs have similar profiles for side effects, even when given in lesser doses, the additive effect may be clinically an adverse one, e.g. the nephrotoxicity of streptomycin and kanamycin. A knowledge of the profiles of side effects of the concurrently administered drugs would alert a clinician to watch for adverse reactions. Sometimes it might be essential to employ sensitive laboratory tests to detect the side effect at subclinical level e.g. basal and serial leucocyte counts would be mandatory when two drugs with potential bone marrow suppressant effects arc being administered concurrently.

Relative Overdosage Toxicity

Drug interaction could lead to a relative overdosage toxicity when one drug converts a safe dose of another drug into a toxic dose by pharmacokinetic or pharmacodynamic mechanisms. Antacids increase the absorption of chloroquine and can be responsible for greater chloroquine toxicity. Hypoglycemia due to a sulphonylurea can be severe when the drug is displaced from the protein bound state by a sulphonamide. Allopurinol, by blocking the metabolism of mercaptopurine, can markedly enhance the toxicity of the latter drug. The example of toxicity of monoamine oxidase inhibitors and pressor amines has been notorious. However, theoretically an Ayurvedic drug can interact with M.A.O. inhibitor. A patient of depression may be receiving a M.A.O. inhibitor. 'Kaunch'-Mucuna pruriens is rich in catecholamine precursors and a severe hypertensive crisis could occur. In India a 'Kounch' reaction may occur instead of a 'cheese reaction'. The oughan allergic reaction is a very complex phenomenon, histamine release does play a significant role in the clinical manifestations of allergy. Drugs known to release histamine e.g. polymeric, tubo-293 curative, etc. can markedly enhance a drug allergic reaction. The drugs inhibiting the biodegradation of histamine can also enhance the histamine mediated effects of drug allergy. Hydralazine inhibits diamante oxidase, the enzyme responsible for oxidative domination of histamine. Chloroquine and a number of other antimalarials drugs inhibit the enzyme imidazole-N-methyltransferase, the other biodegradative enzyme for histamine (Cohn, 1965). Chloroquine and hydralazine can significantly enhance the histamine effects of an allergic drug reaction. More research in this area required.

Increased Secondary Effects

Secondary effects have been defined as the indirect consequence of a primary drug action. Moniliasis or vitamin deficiency following the use of the broad spectrum antibiotics would be such secondary effects. An example of increased secondary effect is exacerbated monilias is when a woman on the oral contraceptive pill also receives tetracyclines. Oral contraceptives, somehow, predispose a patient to monilial infection.

Severe Idiosyncratic Reactions

True idiosyncrasy implies an inherent qualitatively abnormal reaction to a drug. Any sulphonamide and a nitrofuran, if given together, may precipitate a severe hemolysis in a patient with Glucose-6-phosphate dehydrogenase deficiency. This type of drug interaction can also occur in patients with other genetic and enzymic defects. Greater teratogenic effects or additive addiction hazard can occur with drugs having potentially similar hazards or by the effect of one drug on the kinetics of other drug. Lastly, miscellaneous drug interactions would include those phenomena which cannot be classified in any of the aforesaid categories. There have been several interesting reviews on drug interactions and it may not be long before we may also have a Journal devoted fully to drug interactions.

Disease-Drug Interactions

In addition to the drug-drug interactions just discussed, drug-disease interactions can occur. These include interactions between certain drugs and specific disease states. Severe liver disease can be associated with reduced metabolic clearance and higher plasma levels of drugs extensively metabolized by the liver. Although liver disease reduces drug clearance on average, the change is relatively small and usually not clinically relevant except in patients with near terminal liver disease. The effects of renal disease on elimination of drugs that are primarily cleared renally are more predictable and well established guidelines exist for dosage of many drugs in renal disease. Heart failure reduces liver blood flow and causes a reduction in clearance for drugs such as lidocaine or propranolol that are usually extensively cleared by the liver and acute myocardial infarction reduces clearance of some drugs, such as lidocaine, as well. Acute viral infection and changes in thyroid function have been associated with altered clearance for some drugs, such as theophylline and warfarin. However, the results are so variable between individuals that it is difficult to predict who is at risk and these changes are usually only clinically important in cases of extremely impaired organ function.

Table 12.3: Drug-disease interactions

Liver disease
Renal disease
Cardiac disease (hepatic blood flow)
Acute myocardial infarction
Acute viral infection
Hypothyroidism or hyperthyroidism

Food-Drug Interactions

Several drugs are known to interact with foods. One of the early observations was the reduced absorption of tetracycline when taken with milk products. The chelation of tetracycline by calcium prevents it from being absorbed from the intestines. Dietary sources of vitamin K, such as spinach or broccoli, may increase the dosage requirement for warfarin by a pharmacodynamic antagonism of its effect. Patients should be counseled to maintain a consistent diet during warfarin therapy. Grapefruit juice contains a bioflavonoid that inhibits CYP3A and blocks the metabolism of many drugs. This was first described for felodipine but has now been observed with several drugs. This interaction can lead to reduced clearance and higher blood levels when the drugs are taken simultaneously with grapefruit juice. Grapefruit juice (GFJ) is often taken at breakfast in the western countries when drugs are also often taken. GFJ contains bioflavonoids mainly naringin and furacoumarin which cause mechanism based inhibition of presystemic elimination of a number of drugs and increase their bioavailability.

Grapefruit juice, by inhibiting CYP3A4, increases the concentrations of several drugs. This could be clinically relevant especially in older patients or those with liver failure. Although there is an interaction with felodipine, there is no clinically significant effect from the interaction with amlodipine.

Cheese reaction (hyperadrenergic crisis) can occur when a patient on MAO inhibitors consumes cheese of cheese containing preparations e.g. cheese tomato in a marriage party. This is because of tyramine present in cheese, that leads to release of catecholamines in the body. Since the patient is on MAO inhibitors there is already decreased metabolism of catecholamines in the body, hence exaggerated response.

In closing, it is impossible to remember all of the drug interactions that can occur. It is therefore important to develop a stepwise approach to preventing adverse reactions due to drug interactions (Table 12.4).

Table 12.4: Prevention of drug interactions: A stepwise approach

1. ***Take a medication history***
2. ***Remember high risk patients***
• Any patient taking 2 medications
• Anticonvulsants, antibiotics, digoxin, warfarin, amiodarone, etc
3. ***Check pocket reference***
4. ***Consult pharmacists/drug info specialists***
5. ***Check up-to-date computer program***

First, taking a good medication history is essential. The "AVOID Mistakes" mnemonic given in Table 12.5 can help health care practitioners to develop good habits when performing this task.

Second, it is essential that physicians develop an understanding of which patients are at risk for drug

Table 12.5: Points to remember in history taking

A-Allergies
V-Vitamins and herbs
O-Old drugs and OTC
I-Interactions
D-Dependence

interactions. Of course any patient taking 2 medications is at some risk. Studies show that the rate of adverse drug reactions increases exponentially in patients taking 4 or more medications. Importantly, some categories of drugs are especially at high risk for interactions. These categories include anticonvulsants, antibiotics and certain cardiac drugs such as digoxin, warfarin and amiodarone.

Third, any time a patient is taking multiple drugs, we recommend that the first step be to check a readily available pocket reference, recognizing that the interaction may not be listed and a more complete search may be required.

Fourth, consult other members of the health care team. Depending upon the practice setting, this may be a clinical pharmacologist, a hospital pharmacist, a specially trained office staff nurse or the nearby pharmacist in community practice.

Fifth, use one of the computerized databases available. Up-to-date databases are maintained by gsm.com and epocrates.com and others. The latter can be placed on a hand-held computer (e.g. Palm Pilot) and can be configured to automatically update each time you synchronize with the desktop computer. The Medical Letter Drug Interaction Program is inexpensive and updated quarterly.

The list of drug interactions is ever increasing and very soon, for intelligent bedside therapeutics, we may require computer technology providing adequate data storage and quick retrieval of relevant information. For rational and safe therapy, the medical students, the residents and the practising doctors must be made aware of probable drug interactions. An active educational programme, organized by clinical pharmacology divisions in medical colleges, would be of an immense help in cultivating rational therapeutic practice.

CHAPTER THIRTEEN

ADRs Associated with Self-Medication

To feel unwell is very common. The common symptoms experienced in daily life are usually pain, common cold or digestive symptoms. Self-medication is the most common response to above symptoms. A medicine is taken in 50% of above cases. e.g. use of antihistamines for common cold.

Self medication is defined as "use of medicinal products not requiring medical prescription by consumers on their own initiative and responsibility to treat self-recognised disorders or symptoms when they consider such use appropriate".

Self-medication is common in the following conditions:

1. In treatment of uncomplicated chronic recurrent diseases.
2. Reuse of a prescribed medicine by the same person and for the same problem.
3. Reuse of original prescription by a different person or for different problem.

The worldwide market of OTC medicines which presently amounts to US $ 36 billion, may grow by 40% during the next 10 years. The trend is more pronounced in Latin America countries, where OTC market is expected to grow by 70%. OTC drugs are used for self-medication. In USA 80 medicines were labeled as OTC drugs (1980-2000). The drugs which are mainly used as OTC drugs are:

- Antibiotics.
- H_2-antihistamines.
- NSAIDs.

- Oral contraceptives.
- Topical acyclovir.
- Hydrocortisone cream.
- Nicotine-cessation of smoking.

Many traditional/alternative medicines are sold as OTC drugs. Most of these drugs have prescription only status, but still two thirds are available without prescription.

In a WHO survey of 142 countries, 99 responded that most of these products can be bought without prescription. In 39 countries, many traditional medicines are used for self medication.

OTC drugs and self medication may lead to ADRs because of:

- Incorrect self-diagnosis and choice of incorrect therapy.
- Incorrect route of administration.
- Excessively prolonged use.
- Risk of dependence and abuse.
- Food and drug interactions.
- Storage in incorrect conditions.
- Failure to recognise:
  - Contraindications.
  - Interactions.
  - Warnings.
  - Precautions.

People are not able to recognise or report these ADRs. Even medicines that don't need a prescription can cause problems. Vitamins, health food products and herbs (in teas or tablets) may also cause adverse reactions. It is important to tell your doctor and pharmacist if you are using these kinds of products.

There is increased risk of dependence and abuse with these drugs e.g. diazepam, cough syrups, antihistamines. This leads to wasteful public expenditure and increased drug induced diseases. But self-medication is very commonly practiced by people. The reasons are multifactorial depending on the community, some of the reasons are:

- Cost and time of visiting a doctor.
- Overburdened health care system.
- Common believes in the society.
- Worldwide promotional and cross border sale of medicines via internet.

The number of websites for mail order pharmacies were 2,44,546 in 2000.

It is a common belief that self-medication is not a good practice and should be discouraged, but you will be surprised to know that self-medication has important role to play in health care system of a country. With continued improvement in people's education, general knowledge and socioeconomic status, self-medication has been successfully integrated into many health care systems throughout the world. If used appropriately self-medication can take care of health problems of the society very effectively.

WHO has given guidelines (2000) for self-medication. As per these guidelines:

1. Active ingredient at the intended dose should have low inherent toxicity.
2. Intended use should be appropriate for self-medication.
3. Product properties should not have properties that make it undesirable.

   If a new drug the above three basic criteria, the following additional criteria may favour use of the drug as OTC drugs for self medication.
4. Product has been in market for at least 5 years (The withdrawal of most of the products due to ADRs is usually between 3-5 years).
5. The use has been sufficiently extensive or in high enough volume.
6. Adverse events give no cause for concern.

Looking at present scenario it would not be inappropriate to say that oral contraceptives should be available freely from vending machines (real OTC) and cigarettes should be on prescription only (real toxic).

In conclusion we can reiterate that in view of the fact that we are:

- Not using ayurvedic drugs only in the form as described in standard texts making over-the-counter formulations without much heed to the need for individualization.
- Giving ayurvedic drugs in combination with allopathic agents which have a narrow therapeutic margin.
- Using raw plant material that is possibly polluted by environmental and ecological devastation.
- Not having good quality control methodologies.

We must beware. We must not wait for a thalidomide-like tragedy in Ayurveda to shake us out of our complacence that ayurvedic drugs are safe!

Substandard and Counterfeit Drugs

Another factor that can cause adverse drug reactions is the existence on the market of substandard drugs. These are drugs whose composition and ingredients do not meet the correct scientific specifications and which are consequently ineffective and often dangerous to the patient. Substandard products may occur as a result of negligence, human error, insufficient human and financial resources or counterfeiting.

Counterfeit drugs are part of the broader phenomenon of substandard pharmaceuticals. The difference is that they are deliberately and fraudulently mislabeled with respect to identity and/or source. Counterfeiting can apply to both branded and generic products and counterfeit medicines may include products with the correct ingredients but fake packaging, with the wrong ingredients (some of which may be toxic), without active ingredients or with insufficient active ingredients.

In wealthier countries the most frequently counterfeited medicines are new, expensive lifestyle medicines, such as hormones, steroids and antihistamines and recent additions are cholesterol lowering medicines, drugs used for treatment of growth hormone deficiency and for cancer. In developing countries the most counterfeited medicines are those used to treat life-threatening conditions such as malaria, tuberculosis and HIV/AIDS. Antibiotics are also often found among counterfeit medicines.

The Extent of the Problem

The United States Food and Drug Administration (US FDA) estimates that counterfeits make up more than 10% of the global medicines market and are present in both industrialized and developing countries. It is estimated that up to 25% of the medicines consumed in poor countries are counterfeit or substandard. These figures place the annual earnings from the sales of counterfeit and substandard medicines at over US $ 32 billion globally.

Trade in these medicines is more prevalent in countries with weak drug regulation control and enforcement, scarcity and/or erratic supply of basic medicines, unregulated markets and unaffordable prices. However, one of the most counterfeited drugs today is Sildenafil (Viagra), which is sold extensively via the Internet in industrialized countries.

A World Health Organization (WHO) survey of counterfeit medicine reports from 20 countries between January 1999 to October 2000 found that 60% of counterfeit medicine cases occurred in poor countries and 40% in industrialized countries.

In April 1999, reports of 771 cases of substandard medicines had been entered into the WHO database on counterfeits, 77% of which were from developing countries. Data analysis showed that in 60% of the 325 cases an active ingredient was missing from the product. A recent study concluded that up to 40% of artesunate products (the best medicine to combat resistant malaria today) contain no active ingredients and therefore have no therapeutic benefits.

In 2002, GlaxoSmithKline in the United States discovered suspect bottles containing 60 tablets of

Combivir (lamivudine plus zidovudine) that actually contained another medicine, Ziagen (abacavir sulfate). The company determined that counterfeit labels for Combivir tablets were placed on two bottles of Ziagen and labels on another two bottles were suspect. Both medicines are used as part of combination regimens to treat HIV infection and can cause potentially life-threatening hypersensitivity reactions in patients taking other medicines in the combination.

ADRs of Substandard and Counterfeit Medicines

At best, the regular use of substandard or counterfeit medicines leads to therapeutic failure or drug resistance in many cases it can lead to death.

During the meningitis epidemic in Niger in 1995, over 50 000 people were inoculated with fake vaccines, received as a gift from a country which thought they were safe. The exercise resulted in 2,500 deaths. The consumption of paracetamol cough syrup prepared with diethylene glycol (a toxic chemical used in antifreeze) led to 89 deaths in Haiti in 1995 and 30 infant deaths in India in 1998.

Of the one million deaths that occur from malaria annually, as many as 200,000 would be avoidable if the medicines available were effective, of good quality and used correctly. A study conducted in South-East Asia in 2001 revealed that 38% of 104 antimalarial drugs on sale in pharmacies did not contain any active ingredients and had resulted in a number of preventable deaths. In 1999, at least 30 people died in Cambodia after taking counterfeit antimalarials prepared with sulphadoxine-pyrimethamine (an older, less effective antimalarial) which were sold as Artesunate.

Challenges

Because of a lack of regulation and enforcement, the quality, safety and efficacy of both imported and locally manufactured medicines in many developing countries cannot be guaranteed. Subsequently, smuggling and illegal importation of drugs are often rife. Substandard and counterfeit drugs are then not only sold in these countries but also exported or reexported. The situation is worsened by the fact that medicines exported from many industrialized countries are not regulated to the same level as those domestically consumed, while export of drugs to developing countries via free trade zones is increasing. Relabelling of products to mask details of their origin is also known to occur. Some policy makers now believe that drug regulation represents an unnecessary barrier to trade and should be reduced to a minimum. Pharmaceuticals, however, cannot be considered a standard commodity since consumers and prescribers are unable to assess their quality, safety and efficacy and the results can be harmful to patient's health. Growing international and national trade in alternative medicines, including herbal products, is also becoming more complex following rapid increases in demand. Significant quantities of herbal products are now imported by countries in Europe, North America and Asia.

Factors Encouraging Counterfeiting of Drugs

The production of counterfeit drugs need not occur in large infrastructures or facilities. The majority of the counterfeiters apprehended so far carried out their activities in ordinary households, small cottage industries, in backyards or under the shade of a tree. Counterfeiting of medicines is a hugely lucrative business due to high demand and low production costs. The absence of deterrent legislation in many countries also encourages counterfeiters since there is no fear of being apprehended and prosecuted. When prices of medicines are high and price differentials between identical products exist there is a greater incentive for the consumer to seek medicines outside the normal supply system. Poverty, then, is one of the major factors in the production and consumption of substandard products.

CHAPTER FOURTEEN

ADRs Associated with Alternative Medicines

Almost everything discovered in the natural world seems to have been consumed at some time or other as a means of trying alleviate human pain and suffering. There are stories of ADRs with well established allopathic drugs, but herbal drugs pose even a bigger risk and challenge. Worldwide herbal use became popular in 1974, when WHO encouraged developing countries to use traditional plant medicines to fulfill a need unmet by modern systems. 65-80% of the world's population uses traditional medicines mostly plant derived drugs for their primary health needs. For example 70% of western doctors in Japan prescribe kampo drugs daily. As the use of traditional or alternative medicine is increasing, so do reports of ADRs. In China, a country where traditional therapies and products are widely used in parallel with conventional medicines, there were 9854 reported ADRs in 2002 alone, up from 4000 between 1990-1999.

In India situation is worse, over 80% of our population takes ayurvedic medicines either self-prescribed or through a 'Vaidya'. There are more than 1.5 million practitioners of Indian system of medicine (ISM) who use medicinal plants. There are more than 7800 manufacturing units of such medicines in India. "Green medicine" is usually considered safe as compared to allopathic drugs. Affordability and availability also contribute to their wide scale use. International market for these drugs stands at approximately US $ 60 billion per year. Because of long history and usage of these drugs are usually considered harmless. However, they are active drugs and there are reports about their adverse reactions.

Due to aggressive salesmanship and over-the-counter (OTC) availability, these drugs are prescribed by doctors and consumed by patients widely. Patients treated by allopathic medicines simultaneously take ayurvedic medicines, often leading to ADRs. Another point to note is that a large number of herbal preparations are in the market under the label of ayurvedic drugs. Hence, it is obvious, that at least in our country, we have to be aware of salient beneficial and adverse effects of commonly used ayurvedic drugs as much as of allopathic agents.

Ayurvedic drugs that one is likely to encounter in practice can be discussed under two broad categories:

a. The traditional formulations including for example kadhas (decoctions), arishthas (decoctions containing alcohol) or gutis (pills); and
b. The so called ayurvedic formulations which are a combination of different herbal extracts (sometimes aqueous, sometimes alcoholic).

These plants are prescribed individually or together for a particular condition in ayurvedic texts. However, their fixed dose combination, as marketed, may not be mentioned therein. These herbal medicines are prescribed for a wide variety of non-specific conditions like improving vitality, anti-stress effects, boosting immunity and increasing appetite or memory! As we would advise that NSAIDs should not be taken on an empty stomach, Ayurveda gives instructions regarding time of drug administration, the relationship with food, type of food which should be avoided/permitted with the drug etc. The do's and don'ts are clearly there. For example, amalki (amla, *Emblica officinalis*) should be avoided at bedtime to prevent harmful effects on teeth. Ginkgo biloba is used very frequently to prevent vascular disease and increase blood circulation. WHO monitoring centre reported seven cases of excessive bleeding encountered during a surgical operation. Chyavanprash contains large quantities of amla, one wonders whether the package insert with any Chyavanprash mentions this precaution! Similarly, pippali (*Piper longum*) used in asthma should be avoided in patients with peptic ulcer disease and should be consumed with milk. Tribhuvankirti is a combination of several plants which is very commonly used to treat a "cold in the head" and fever. There are clear instructions in Ayurveda that because it contains aconite it should be used cautiously. When used, it should be taken with tulsi (holy basil) juice, ginger juice or honey.

Guggul is derived from the resin of *Commiphora mukul* and is used in a variety of diseases including hypercholesterolemia (in fact gugglulip has been introduced into the market for this condition) and arthritis. Ayurveda specifies that guggul should be used cautiously in patients with peptic ulcer disease. Patient on guggul therapy is advised to avoid sour food, alcohol and heavy exercise. Guggul can be excreted in breast milk and its bitter taste may result in refusal of a breast feed by baby. Trikatu has been reported to cause burning of eyes, palms, and soles. Allergic skin reaction can occur with Lakshmi Vilas Ras. Ginseng, a popular tonic, contains oestrogenic substances which causes gynecomastia and Ginseng abuse syndrome. Some of the ayurvedic formulations which contain bhasmas or metals could cause serious systemic toxicity. St John's Wort an herbal antidepressant has been reported to decrease levels of warfarin by induction of 2C9. A drug interaction between phenytoin and an ayurvedic formulation has also been reported the mechanisms of the adverse reactions with ayurvedic medicines are probably similar to synthetic chemicals. There is also a reported case of breakthrough seizures on account of interaction between phenytoin and an ayurvedic preparation "Shankhapushpi"

Drug Interactions with Herbal Drugs

Another cause of concern with the use of alternative medicine is drug interactions. It has been reported that 70% of patients do not reveal their herbal use to their allopathic practitioners. It is likely that many drug-herbal

Table 14.1: ADRs reported with some herbal drugs

ADR	*Causative drug*
Hepatotoxicity	Chinese herbal teas, Echinacea, germander, chaparral, comfrey
Nausea/vomiting chaparral,	Dandelion, garlic, ginseng, ginkgo
Diarrhoea	Herbal teas, aloe, ligustrum, dandelion, prunelia, garlic, ginseng
Anticoagulant/ antiplatelet	Yarrow, red clover, tang-kuel, salvla
Nervousness, agitation, mood changes, depression, headache, mania	Ginseng
Cholinergic toxicity	Jimson weed
Hallucinogenic	Catnip, kava kava, khat, lobelia, mandrake, nutmeg, jimson weed, yohimbe
Sedation	Peony, salvla, tang-kuel
Seizures, psychosis	Ephedra
Pulmonary hypertension	Chinese herbal teas
Contact dermatitis	Propolis, garlic, Echinacea
Systemic lupus erythematous	Alfalfa
Gynacomastia, vaginal bleeding, mastalgia	Ginseng
Thyroid abnormalities	Kelp, garlic
Hypoglycemia	Atraclylodes, scrufularia, lyceum
Diuresis	Astragalus, peony, dandelion
Hypertension	Licorice, ginseng, ephedra
Hypotension	Astragalus, codonopsis, prunella, scrofularia
Bleeding	Feverfew, garlic, ginkgo, ginger, ginseng
Allergic reactions	Chamomile, feverfew
Photosensitivity	St John Wort

interactions exist but have not yet been detected. It is therefore important that health care providers obtain a complete drug history that includes herbal remedies and other natural products and dietary supplements and that they be alert to potential interactions.

The reasons herbal drugs are prone to cause drug interactions are:

1. These products are mutiingredient formulations.
2. There is usually incomplete information about active principle in the formulation.
3. These drugs are available without prescription (OTC drugs).
4. Herbal and allopathic drugs are taken together by patients.
5. There are 29 official languages in India, hence reporting of ADR language differs.
6. Sometimes herbal and allopathic drugs are present in same formulation e.g. Ginseng+ferrous sulphate.
7. There is no safety information on the labels.

Eucalyptus can induce microsomal liver enzymes while flavonoids from Echinacea purpurea can inhibit CYP450 3A4 isoenzyme. Ingestion of St. John's wort has resulted in several clinically significant interactions with drugs that are metabolized by CYP1A2 or CYP3A including indinavir and cyclosporine. An interaction with digoxin has also been reported that may be mediated by interference with P-glycoprotein, a transport system that pumps drugs across membranes. These interactions are most likely due to induction of the cytochrome P_{450} isozyme or the drug transporter and have caused decreased plasma concentrations of prescription drugs. In the case of cyclosporin, subtherapeutic levels resulted in transplant organ rejection. Warnings about St. John's Wort drug interactions have been extended to oral contraceptives, with labeling suggesting the possibility of breakthrough bleeding and potential for loss of contraceptive effect.

Some Ayurvedic physicians prescribe certain parts of the castor plant Ricinus communis to patients with rheumatoid arthritis. If the patient is also taking other antiarthritic drugs with known gastro-intestinal side effects, the enhanced side effect due to castor plant can be severe. The possibility of enhanced side effects due to concomitant administration of Ayurvedic and modern drugs must be borne in mind.

Table 14.2: Drug interactions of alternative medicines

Allopathic drug	*Alternative medicine*	*ADR*
Alprazolam	Kava	Excessive sedation
Corticosteroids cyclosporine	Echinacea, vitamin E, alfalfa, licorice, astragalus, zinc	Decreases immunosuppressant action
Digoxin	Hawthorn Licorice Uzara root	Potentiates digoxin Hypokalemia Additive cardiac action
Diuretics	Dandelion, uvaursi, goldenseal, agrominoy, burdock, dandelion, juniper, Gossypol	Nullify antihypertensive action, hypokalemia
Hypoglycemic	Chromium, karela	Hypoglycemia
Levothyroxine	Kelp, horseradish	Antagonises action
NSAIDs	Uva-ursi, gossypol	Additive GIT toxicity
MAO inhibitors	Ginseng, yohimbine, ephedra St John Wort	Insomnia, headache Additive action
Phenytoin phenobarbitone	Wormwood, sage, evening primorose oil, borage Shankapushpi	Lower seizure threshold Decreases effect of phenytoin
Spironolactone	Licorice	Decreases effect
Warfarin	Garlic, ginger, ginkgo, feverfew Ginseng	Augments action Decreases effect

Over 90% of pain clinics in UK and 70% in Germany include acupuncture as a form of treatment. A study in Norway reported cases of pneumothorax caused by unqualified acupuncturists. There are also reports of paralysis caused by unqualified manual therapies.

With increase in demand and use of traditional medicines physicians are expected to encounter more ADRs related with these drugs in general practice.

CHAPTER FIFTEEN

Minimizing ADRs

The much publicised withdrawal of rofecoxib and the subsequent doubts about the safety of celecoxib evoked a huge response in both the lay and the medical press. Medical journals have thundered about the irresponsibility of the pharmaceutical industry and the lack of vigilance on the part of government agencies. These criticisms are generally justified, but the. use of new drugs is not solely determined by industry and government. Doctors and patients and community is also responsible to some extent. Efforts at all levels are required to reduce the incidence of preventable ADRs with drugs.

Adverse drug reactions can be minimized by an attending doctor only if he or she has update knowledge about ADRs, the knowledge to drug prescription, the monitoring of drug adverse reaction and to remain vigilant to recognise and record newer adverse reaction that has not been previously recognized. The physician would like to prevent, detect early and treat successfully adverse reactions. Avoidable ADRs can be reduced by more skillful prescribing and this means that doctors must find time to better understand drugs as well as to understand their patients and their diseases.

Patient's Perspective

Tell each of your doctors (if you see more than one) about all of the drugs you are taking, even if you take something for only a short time. You should try to use only one drug store so your pharmacists get to know you and the medicines you take. Pharmacists are trained to look at the drugs you are taking to see whether they might cause an adverse drug reaction. Even medicines that donot need a prescription (OTC medicines) can cause problems. Vitamins, health food products and herbs (in teas or tablets) may also cause adverse reactions. It's important to tell your doctor and pharmacist if you are using these kinds of products.

The following are some adverse drug reactions that you might notice:
- Skin rash.
- Easy bruising.
- Bleeding.
- Severe nausea and vomiting.
- Diarrhea.
- Constipation.
- Confusion.
- Breathing difficulties.

The following are some adverse reactions your doctor might notice during a check-up:
- Changes in laboratory test results.
- Abnormal heartbeat.

Doctor's Perspective

To update the knowledge about the routinely used drugs, physicians must cut down the battalion of drugs being prescribed and the restrict the number of drugs. He or she must have complete and authentic knowledge about adverse effects of drugs being used. Adverse effect may be unwanted effect due to augmented pharmacological drug effect which are dose dependant or bizarre idiosyncratic drug reaction due to genetic susceptibility or immuno-mechanisms. The former are frequent and relatively less serious. The latter are infrequent and usually serious with fatal out come. The former type of reaction in generally attributable to excessive dosage and sometimes due to doctor's negligence. Many a times the drug dosage variation (which may be appropriate for patients in west, may actually not be so for Indians) may be the culprit, especially when a new drug is launched. This may be true for certain drugs, which need strict observation e.g. analgesics and anaesthetics. Thus it is better to use lower drug dosage especially when using newer drugs, but this does not apply to antimicrobials and as drug resistance is likely to reduce the drug efficacy.

Both patient and doctor's perspective can be taken care of, if an effective programme is developed towards this end having following components:

1. A reliable source of information.
2. A sound prescribing policy.
3. A monitoring system.
4. Some methods of identifying new, and previously unrecognized adverse reactions, and
5. Research to investigate cause and risk factors.

These are essential components of any programme targeted to reduce ADRs.

Source of Drug Information

Although pharma houses provide knowledge about the drug and their hazardous events that may occur during their use in therapeutic indications with recommended dosage the information given by these houses is often incomplete and hence the data loses its reliability. There should be a pooled information given by drug safety committee to be backed by WHO and a regular update must appear especially on the adverse effect of newer drugs in the leading medical journals, so that physicians remain comprehensively updated to face any eventuality.

The typical example of how the information provided can change the concepts and beliefs of the patients, doctors and community is information on new selective COX-2 inhibitor NSAIDs. These drugs were promoted as safer to GIT as compared to non-selective COX NSAIDs. In 1999 it was known that the main demonstrated effect of COX-2s, compared with NSAIDs, was a reduction in shallow 'endoscopic' ulcers which are clinically unimportant. The beneficial effect on serious, complicated ulcers was very much less. In patients with rheumatoid arthritis and no other risk factors, the annual risk of developing a complication related to

NSAID use is only 0.4%. COX-2s could possibly reduce this to 0.2% (likely to be expressed as a 50% reduction for marketing purposes).

Many doctors also gained the false impression that selective drugs were also less likely than conventional NSAIDs to have adverse effects on blood pressure and the kidneys. This view was also held by some key opinion leaders, people who always have a major influence on prescribing patterns and, for this reason, are invited by pharmaceutical companies to talk to groups of prescribers. To complicate the situation, the media persuaded consumers that the new 'wonder' drugs were more efficacious than older medications. Word of mouth completed a marketer's dream situation. Certainly the drugs were heavily promoted by both industry and the media, but why did prescribers fail to follow ethical principles? The facts were all there in many independent sources of information. Cox-2 inhibitors are either being banned (nimesulide) or withdrawn voluntary by manufacturer (rofecoxib).

There is no merit in being among the first to prescribe a new drug whatever the pressures from patients and drug companies. It has been well said that 'For all newly licensed drugs, confidence about safety can only be provisional. It is essential that both prescribers and consumers grasp this fundamental fact.

There seems to be a glamour about anything new, despite the absence of long term safety information when a drug is first approved. Of course the industry designs and interprets trials to maximise favourable commercial outcomes. Of course it puts the best possible spin on its marketing messages, but doctors should be smart enough to see through the hype created. They need to know that when a drug first appears on the market only limited safety data are available and long term outcomes, both good and bad, can only emerge with time and appropriately designed, prospective safety studies. It is well established that most prescribers obtain the majority of their information from the pharmaceutical industry and they therefore need more training in how to evaluate the information and what questions to ask drug representatives.

How Doctors Can Get Updated About Drugs?

Knowledge and ideas about drugs are constantly changing. More and more new drugs are coming on the market. New experience with existing drugs is expanding (side effects, new indications/ways of using). A physician is expected to know about new developments in drug therapy. However in many parts of the world, objective and unbiased information about drugs is a luxury which is difficult for most of the physicians to access. It is difficult for busy physicians to have satisfactory knowledge of all these drugs. Hence, selection and use of right drug in an appropriate manner becomes a challenge.

How you can keep up-to-date about drug information in spite of your busy schedule?

The Sources of Information Are

1. Written form-journals, reference books, drug bulletins.
2. Verbally-through discussions in meetings, journal clubs in institutions.
3. Tape/video/online-journals, CDs.
4. Drug Information Centers.
5. Pharmaceutical industry.
6. Internet.

Written forms which can be used are:

1. Drug compendia-these list the drugs available on the market.
2. Drug bulletins.
3. Medical journals.
4. National list of essential drugs and standard treatment guidelines.
5. General Pharmacological reference- Goodman and Gilman's: The Pharmacological basis of Therapeutics.

6. Martindale's The extra Pharmacopoeia-excellent reference book, gives all information on all chemicals used with references.
7. Avery' drug treatment-more specialised.
8. Meyler's side effects of drugs.
9. MIMS-monthly index of medical specialties-these provide information on:
   - Generic/brand names.
   - Chemical composition.
   - Indications/contraindications.
   - Side effects, interactions.
   - Price.

10. Drug bulletins are preferred because they are:
    - Critical source of new drug information.
    - Promote rational drug therapy.
    - Appear at frequent intervals.
    - Sponsors-government agencies, university departments, professional bodies, non-industry sponsored.

    Some drug bulletins available In India are:
    Drug bulletin-PGI.
    Australian prescriber is available free of charge.
    Others are: Drugs and therapeutic bulletin (UK), Medical letter (USA).
11. Journals
    The important ones are: The Lancet, New England Journal of Medicine, British Medical Journal. Tons of information is available in these journals. Thousands are published and they vary enormously in quality.
    - Only a small proportion publish scientifically validated articles.
    - Good journal are peer reviewed by independent experts, usually no advertisements are there.
    - Define range of drugs available to prescriber.
    - Consensus on the treatment of choice for the most common diseases and complaints.
    - Index Medicus has list of major reputable journals.
12. Symposia/conferences
    Symposia are useful for disseminating information. The objective scientific content of such

meetings should be paramount, and presentations by independent scientists and health professionals are helpful to this end.

13. DIC (Drug Information Centre)
    - Very useful.
    - Prescribers and general public can call.
    - Use reference books online.

    Examples:
    - DIC-Philippines-Dept. of Pharmacology.
    - DIC-Kathmandu, Nepal:
      –2 clinical pharmacologists.
      –1 Pharmacist.
14. Pharmaceutical Industry

    Pharmaceutical Industry has multi-track approach for providing information to physicians. This is the commonest source of drug information for physicians and available through all channels of communication i.e. verbal, written and computerised. These channels includes professional meeting, advertising in journals, direct mailing, medical representatives etc.

    15-20% of budget of a pharmaceutical industry is for promotion of products. Out of those > 50% is spent on medical representatives. 90% of the physicians see medical representatives. This is the easiest way to gather new drug information. A substantial percentage of physicians heavily rely on representatives as source of information about drugs. But, it has been observed that these representatives emphasize only the positive aspects of products and overlook or give little coverage to the negative aspects (ADRs). Most of the information is commercially driven.

    Should You Avoid Representatives?

    Medical representatives are criticized a lot, but there network is very huge and now they have become an integral part of medical infrastructure in the country. Hence make best use of this huge network for getting drug information in a desirable way! Ask about publication of drug safety in an authentic journal. Optimize the time spent with medical representatives. Remember following points while dealing with a representative:

- Take control of the discussion.
- You get the information you need.
- Ask for officially registered drug information and compare it with what industry has got printed.
- Comparison with standard treatment used.
- Particularly look for side effects and contra-indications.
- Ask for published references on efficacy and safety.
- If it is 'me too' drug (analogue of same class e.g. new proton pump inhibitor) ask about price.
- Do not start by using free samples on a few patients or family members.
- Do not base your conclusions on the treatment of a few patients.

15. Internet

Adverse effects are the prime health hazards of prescription drugs. In order to manage an adverse drug reaction it is important to be aware of all possible drug reactions and drug interactions. However, given the current scenario of introduction of new drugs into market, it is impossible to keep track of all reports of reactions. This is where the web comes to the rescue. Internet is another source of drug information, but all the information available is not authentic. Check the authenticity of the website.

Advantages:

- A large number of sources.
- Quick and easy.

Disadvantages:

- Illegal advertising and complaints have increased.
- Use catchy slogans e.g. Scientific breakthrough, miraculous cure, secret formula, ancient ingredients, antiageing, all natural.

- Use case histories of successful consumers, authenticity of whom is questionable.

Keeping up-to-date should not be too difficult for physicians in developed countries, but it can be far from easy in some parts of the world where access to independent sources of drug information is very limited. But wherever you live and work it is important to develop a strategy to maximize your access to key information you need for optimal benefit of the drugs you prescribe.

Rational Use of Drugs (RUD)

ADRs can be reduced significantly by rational use of drugs. Rational use of drugs is defined as "patients receive drugs appropriate to their clinical needs, in doses that meet their own individual requirements, for an adequate period of time and at the lowest cost to them and their community"

The following simple guidelines will help rational use of drugs:

1. Appropriate indication.
2. Appropriate drug.
3. Appropriate dosage, duration and route of administration.
4. Appropriate patient.
5. Appropriate patient information.
6. Appropriate monitoring.
7. Appropriate cost.

Why irrational treatment common? Worldwide more than 50% of all medicines are prescribed, dispensed or sold inappropriately, while 50% patients fail to take them correctly. The reasons for irrational use of drugs are:

a. Polypharmacy.
b. Use of drugs in inadequate dosage and conditions e.g. antibiotic for diarrhoea.
c. Over use of injections e.g. multivitamins.
d. Inappropriate self-medication e.g. tonics for malnutrition.
e. Use of expensive drugs unnecessarily e.g. use of third generation cephalosporin when a first-line, narrow spectrum antimicrobial is indicated.

Irrational use of drugs is a common cause for increased ADRs due to various reasons e.g. drug interactions, development of resistance, transmission of HIV/ AIDS hepatitis etc.

The essential components of RUD includes:

1. Essential drug list.
2. Rational prescribing.
3. Information to doctors.
4. Information to patients.
5. Quality assurance.

Rational drug use provides therapeutically sound treatment with less ADRs and drug interactions.

Essential drug list (List is given in last chapter, Table 19.10): Essential medicines are those that satisfy the priority health care needs of the population and available at all times in adequate amounts in the appropriate dosage forms with assured quality. Selection criteria includes due regard to disease prevalence, evidence on efficacy and safety and comparative cost-effectiveness.

Evidently, the word "Essential" does not purport to convey that number of other drugs available in the market are non-essential. WHO has a list of essential drugs that can be used as a guide to construct national list of essential drugs.

If this list is used then following advantages a physician can get:

1. Training more focused and therefore easier.
2. More experience with fewer drugs. It is recommended that do not use a new drug in general practice if it less than 5 years old in market.
3. Focused drug information.
4. Better recognition of ADRs.
5. Less costly drugs are prescribed.

The process of rational treatment can be followed in a sequential manner as given in figure 15.1.

Define patient's problem
↓
Specify therapeutic objective
↓
Verify suitability of your selected drug/treatment
↓
Start treatment
↓
Give information, instructions and warnings about drug/treatment
↓
Monitor treatment

Fig. 15.1: Rational treatment

There should be policy at national levels to reinforce the concept of rational use of drugs. National policy on the safe and appropriate (rational) use of drugs should contain:

- Undergraduate and continuing education on rational use of drugs.
- Assessment of pharmacotherapy practices.
- Promotion of rational use of drugs.
- Preparing and distribution of educational and informational materials.
- Monitoring and evaluation of activities.

Drugs are not testes in special population groups like elderly, children and pregnancy, hence be cautious while prescribing for these patients.

Elderly and ADRs

Very old are very young patients are more prone to ADRs It is estimated that by the year 2020 elderly people will constitute 11-12% of total population. Variations occur in pharmacokinetics and pharmacodynamic with age. Older people usually use multiple drugs. Variation is response and polypharmacy is because of ageing itself and common age related diseases. Multiple drugs and variation in response expose the elderly to more ADRs. To prevent ADRs in elderly the common principles are:

a. Start slow, go slow.
b. One drug, one dose.

c. Start at right time, stop at right time.
d. Avoid certain drugs.

Children and ADRs

Pharmacokinetics of drugs are variable in children. Bioavailability of rifampicin, gentamicin, phenytoin, phenobarbitone and acetaminophen is increased in children. There is limited capacity for metabolism in newborn and decreased elimination is seen for most of the drugs. Phase 2 reactions are not well developed. Similarly pharmacodynamic vary in children. Nimesulide is hepatotoxic in children, but still used in our country for children. Safer antipyretics like paracetamol is available. Similarly ciprofloxacin can lead to tendon damage and rupture and it is not recommended for children, but in our country there is no restriction for its use in children. In children few precautions are a must:

- Always calculate the appropriate dose for the age of the child.
- Do not use newer drugs, use only well established drugs.
- Avoid polytherapy.

Pregnancy, Lactation and ADRs

In pregnant state pharmacokinetics and pharmacodynamic of a drug changes, hence predisposes a pregnant female to ADRs. Thalidomide is a classical example of teratogenic effects. It was synthesized in 1954 in Germany and four years later was marketed as sedative. It was widely used by pregnant females for nausea and vomiting. It was considered safe because in toxicity studies in rodents , it did not produce any toxic effect. Thalidomide led to birth of babies with seal like limbs (phocomelia). It is estimated that approximately 20,000 babies suffered toxicity of thalidomide. It was withdrawn in 1961. It is recommended that no drug should be given in its trimester of pregnancy.

FDA has classified drugs and risks in pregnancy as per Table 15.1

Table 15.1: Categories of risk in pregnancy

Category	*Interpretation*	*Examples*
A	Adequate, well-controlled studies in pregnant women have not shown an increased risk of fetal abnormalities to the fetus in any trimester of pregnancy.	Folic acid Thyroxine
B	Animal studies have revealed no evidence of harm to the fetus, however, there are no adequate and well-controlled studies in pregnant women. **OR** Animal studies have shown an adverse effect, but adequate and well-controlled studies in pregnant women have failed to demonstrate a risk to the fetus in any trimester.	Amoxycillin Paracetamol Lignocaine Cefaclor Famotidine Lansoprazole Hydrochloro-thiazide
C	Animal studies have shown an adverse effect and there are no adequate and well-controlled studies in pregnant women. **OR** No animal studies have been conducted and there are no adequate and well-controlled studies in pregnant women.	Morphine Atropine Adrenaline Thiopentone Felodipine Furosemide
D	Adequate well-controlled or observational studies in pregnant women have demonstrated a risk to the fetus. However, the benefits of therapy may outweigh the potential risk. For example, the drug may be acceptable if needed in a life-threatening situation or serious disease for which safer drugs cannot be used or are ineffective.	Aspirin Aspirin Carbamazepine Lorazepam Doxycycline Imipramine Lithium
X	Adequate well-controlled or observational studies in animals or pregnant women have demonstrated positive evidence of fetal abnormalities or risks. The use of the product is contraindicated in women who are or may become pregnant.	Isotretinoin Ergometrine Estrogens Lovastatin Iodine- 125

The commonly used drugs during pregnancy are:

- Non-narcotic analgesics: Paracetamol is drug of choice.
- Antibacterial agents.
- Antacids: Safe in second and third trimester.
- Drugs for nausea/ vomiting: Often unrewarding, probably best of a fairly ineffective range of options.

Assess the benefit/risk ratio for the condition being treated.

Care should be taken while prescribing drugs to lactating mothers. Drugs may be classified as per the following criteria:

a. Drugs undetected in breast milk: aminoglycosides.
b. Drugs reach the baby but insignificant dose: non-narcotic analgesics, penicillin.
c. Drugs reach the baby with significant dose: aspirin, benzodiazepines, barbiturates, tetracyclines, carbimazole.

The following principles should be followed when prescribing for breastfeeding mothers:

- Avoid unnecessary drug use and limit use of over-the-counter (OTC) products.
- Breastfeeding mothers should seek advice on the suitability of OTC products.
- Avoid use of drugs known to cause serious toxicity in adults or children.
- Neonates (and particularly premature infants) are at greater risk from exposure to drugs via breast milk, because of immature excretory functions and the consequent risk of drug accumulation.
- Choose a regimen and route of administration which presents the minimum amount of drug to the infant.
- It is best to avoid long-acting preparations, especially those of drugs likely to cause serious side effects (e.g. antipsychotic agents).
- Multiple drug regimens may pose an increased risk especially when adverse effects such as drowsiness are additive.
- Infants exposed to drugs via breast milk should be monitored for unusual signs or symptoms.

- Avoid new drugs if a therapeutically equivalent alternative that has been more widely used is available. A robust assessment of the balance of benefit to risk requires data both on the drug's passage into breast milk and its effects in infants: there is rarely enough information available for new drugs to allow such an assessment to be made.
- Assess the benefit/risk ratio for both mother and infant.

Ethical Criteria for Drug Promotion

WHO has formulated ethical criteria for medicinal drug promotion. The main objective of ethical criteria for medicinal drug promotion is to support and encourage the improvement of health care through the rational use of medicinal drugs. The essential features of are:

1. Ethical criteria for drug promotion provides the foundation for proper behaviour concerning the promotion of medicinal drugs, consistent with the search for truthfulness and righteousness. These criteria constitute general principles for ethical standards which could be adapted by governments to national circumstances as appropriate to their political, economic, cultural, social, educational, scientific and technical situation, laws and regulations, disease profile, therapeutic traditions and the level of development of their health system. They apply to prescription and non-prescription medicinal drugs ("over-the-counter drugs"). They also apply generally to traditional medicines as appropriate, and to any other product promoted as a medicine.
2. "Promotion" refers to all informational and persuasive activities by manufacturers and distributors, the effect of which is to induce the prescription, supply, purchase and/or use of medicinal drugs. All promotion making claims concerning medicinal drugs should be reliable, accurate, truthful, informative, balanced, up-to-date, capable of substantiation and in good taste. They should not contain misleading or unverifiable statements or omissions likely to induce medically unjustifiable drug use or to give rise to

undue risks. The word "safe" should only be used if properly qualified. Comparison of products should be factual, fair and capable of substantiation. Scientific data in the public domain should be made available to prescribers and any other person entitled to receive it, on request, as appropriate to their requirements. Scientific and educational activities should not be deliberately used for promotional purposes.

3. Information that such advertisements should usually contain, among others includes:
   - The name(s) of the active ingredient(s) using either international nonproprietary names (INN) or the approved generic name of the drug.
   - Brand name.
   - Content of active ingredient(s) per dosage form or regimen.
   - Name of other ingredients known to cause problems.
   - Approved therapeutic uses.
   - Dosage form or regimen.
   - Side-effects and major adverse drug reactions.
   - Precautions, contra-indications and warnings.
   - Major interactions.
   - Name and address of manufacturer or distributor.
   - Reference to scientific literature as appropriate.
4. To fight drug addiction and dependency, scheduled narcotic and psychotropic drugs should not be advertised to the general public. While health education aimed at children is highly desirable, drug advertisements should not be directed at children.
5. Medical representatives should have an appropriate educational background. They should be adequately trained. They should possess sufficient medical and technical knowledge and integrity to present information on products and carry out other promotional activities in an accurate and responsible manner. Exposure of medical representatives and trainees to feedback from the medical and allied professions and from independent members of the public, particularly regarding risks, can be salutary. Medical

representatives should make available to prescribers and dispensers complete and unbiased information for each product discussed, such as an approved scientific data sheet or other source of information with similar content.

6. Free samples of legally available prescription drugs may be provided in modest quantities to prescribers, generally on request. Free samples of non-prescription drugs to the general public for promotional purposes.
7. Postmarketing scientific studies and surveillance should not be misused as a disguised form of promotion.
8. Appropriate information being important to ensure the rational use of drugs, all packaging and labeling material should provide information consistent with that approved by the country's drug regulatory authority. Adequate information on the use of medicinal drugs should be made available to patients.

A Good Medication History can AVOID mistakes. Remember following points while taking history:

- Allergies.
- Vitamins and herbs.
- Old drugs and OTC ... as well as current.
- Interactions.
- Dependence.

A history of allergies or previous history of adverse reactions to any drugs should be elicited in a way that will yield the most useful information. For example, rather than asking about a history of drug allergy, the patient should be asked whether there is any drug that should not be prescribed for any reason. A specific question should be asked about the use of vitamins and herbal or other natural products. Old drugs (prescription and over the counter) should be considered as well as new drugs, since some of the effects (either toxicity or potential for drug interactions) could be relatively long lasting. The potential for adverse drug interactions should be evaluated. The need for a behavioral contract between the physician and the patient should be considered in an effort to help the patient reach the therapeutic goal, either in the case of drug dependence or adherence to a therapeutic regimen, with a clear plan. Finally, a family history of benefits or problems with any medications will help determine whether pharmacogenetics should be considered in tailoring drug therapy.

How to Recognize ADRs

Since ADRs may occur through the same physiological and pathological pathways as different diseases, they are difficult and sometimes impossible to distinguish. However, the following step-wise approach may be helpful in assessing possible drug-related ADRs:

1. Ensure that the medicine ordered is the medicine received and actually taken by the patient at the dose advised.
2. Verify that the onset of the suspected ADR was after the drug was taken, not before and discuss carefully the observation made by the patient.
3. Determine the time interval between the beginning of drug treatment and the onset of the event.
4. Evaluate the suspected ADR after discontinuing the drugs or reducing the dose and monitor the patient's status. If appropriate, restart the drug treatment and monitor recurrence of any adverse events (dechallenge and rechallenge).
5. Analyse the alternative causes (other than the drug) that could on their own have caused the reaction.
6. Use relevant up-to-date literature and personal experience as a health professional on drugs and their ADRs and verify if there are previous conclusive reports on this reaction. The National Pharmacovigilance Centre and Drug Information Centers are very important resources for obtaining information on ADR. The manufacturer of the drug can also be a resource to consult.
7. Report any suspected ADR to the person nominated for ADR reporting in the hospital or directly to the National ADR Centre.

What Should Be Reported?

- For "new" drugs—report all suspected reactions, including minor ones. (In many countries drugs are still considered "new" up to five years after marketing authorization).
- For established or well-known drugs—report all serious or unexpected (unusual) suspected ADRs.
- Report if an increased frequency of a given reaction is observed.
- Report all suspected ADRs associated with drug-drug, drug-food or drug-food supplements (including herbal and complementary products) interactions.
- Report ADRs in special fields of interest such as drug abuse and drug use in pregnancy and during lactation.
- Report when suspected ADRs are associated with drug withdrawals.
- Report ADRs occurring from overdose or medication error.
- Report when there is a lack of efficacy or when suspected pharmaceutical defects are observed.

Thus, report all suspected adverse reactions that you consider of clinical importance as soon as possible.

How to Report ADRs?

Local Case Report Forms (CRF) should be obtained from the National Drug Regulatory Authority. Some countries have included CRF in their National Formularies (British National Formulary, Formularies of South Africa, Zimbabwe etc.). There are different Case Report Forms in different countries. But all of them have at least four sections (Fig. 15.2) which should be completed.

Health care providers have misconceptions about reporting ADRs. These misconceptions include the ideas that:

1. All serious ADRs are documented by the time a drug is marketed.
2. It is hard to determine if a drug is responsible for the ADR.

Sample ADR format

1. Patient information
    - Patient identifier ______________________
    - Age at time of event or date of birth________
    - Gender________
    - Weight________
2. Adverse event or product
    - Problem date of event date of this report
    - Description of event or problem
    - Relevant tests/laboratory data (if available)
    - Other relevant patient information/history
    - Outcomes attributed to adverse event
3. Suspected medication(s)
    - Name (INN and brand name) dose frequency route used
    - Therapy date
    - Diagnosis for use
    - Event abated after use stopped or dose reduced
    - Batch number Expiration date
    - Event reappeared after
    - Reintroduction of the treatment
    - Concomitant medical products and therapy dates
4. Reporter
    - Name, address and telephone number
    - Speciality and occupation

Fig. 15.2: Sample ADR format

3. ADRs should only be reported if absolute certainty exists that the ADR is related to a particular drug; and finally.
4. One case reported by an individual physician does not contribute to medical knowledge.

Let's discuss each misconception and clarify doubts:

1. As we have seen, rare ADRs are usually not documented by the time a drug is marketed.
2. It can be hard to determine if an individual drug caused a reaction in a complicated patient receiving multiple medications. However, the temporal relationship of a reaction with regard to the administration

of a new drug can be helpful. Also, biological plausibility (asking if the drug's mechanism of action makes this possible or likely) can also be helpful. The bottom line is, even when in doubt about whether a drug caused the reaction, report it.

3. A suspicion of an adverse drug reaction should be reported. A health care provider does not have to be absolutely certain that a drug caused a reaction. All reports contribute to the heightening of the awareness of FDA safety scientists as they monitor all of the evidence to evaluate the potential for drug-related toxicity.
4. One individual report can make a difference. Many drug withdrawals began with one clinical report that initiated further investigation. In the example case in this module, a single report ultimately led to the removal of terfenadine from the market. This report potentially saved many lives and led to a better understanding of the mechanism involved in causing torsades de pointes. Almost all drugs are now evaluated prior to being released on the market for their potential to induce cardiac arrhythmias, also as a result of this single case report.

There are many examples of the importance of ADRs reporting in the improvement of information in labeling of many effective pharmaceutical products (new possible ADRs, contraindications, dosage etc.). Cyclophosphamide has been on the market for several years in many countries. In January 2001 there were some new reactions included in the labels: Stevens Johnson syndrome and toxic epidermal necrolysis.

The following aspects of labelling and package inserts should be considered:

- Consumer information which is simple and not confusing.
- Indication of the item as a medicinal product.
- Composition of the product including international nonproprietary name (INN)/generic name of the active substance.

- Uses for which the product is intended.
- Mode of use, including route of administration (systemic or local), maximum single dose, maximum daily dose and duration of treatment.
- The product is intended for (children or adults).
- Presentation of the most important precautions, contraindications and adverse effects clearly stated in easily understandable language.
- Specific warnings and information for use during pregnancy, lactation, by the elderly or in patients with renal or hepatic failure.
- When medical advice should be sought.
- Duration of use.
- Information on storage conditions and shelf-life.
- Inactive ingredients listed.
- Expected benefit when the drug is used properly.
- The use of pictograms.

Some drugs/substances are covered under various schedules of Drugs and Cosmetics act, 1940. Some important schedules on labeling are:

Schedule H-List of substances that could be dispensed only on the prescription of a registered medical practitioner e.g. antibiotics, diazepam.

Schedule G-List of substances that are required to be used only under medical supervision e.g. insulin, antihistamines.

Systems Interventions and Their Limitations

- Systems interventions
  - Electronic prescription entry and bar-coding.
  - Computerized medication records.
  - Drug interaction software.
- Limitations
  - Fragmented healthcare delivery and prescription filling.
  - Information not uniformly translated into practice.
- Message
  - Can't rely completely on technology.

- Need basic knowledge of clinical pharmacology of drug interactions.

Recent research have shown that many adverse drug reactions can be prevented and detected through the use of systems interventions. For example, many health systems have instituted new technologies to minimize patient injury due to medication errors and drug-drug interactions. Tools like computerized physician order and prescription entry and bar coding systems have demonstrated tangible benefits. The potential for reducing medication errors by using computerized medical records as well as drug-interaction screening software that detects and alerts the physician and/or pharmacist to potentially serious drug interactions has been recognized.

These technological solutions do have limitations, however. The fragmentation of healthcare delivery may result in incomplete records. More significant is the fact that, although this information is available, it is not uniformly or optimally incorporated into decision making. This is exemplified in the example that pharmacists filled prescriptions for drug combinations that were known to interact even though computerized drug interaction software was in place.

These findings should reinforce the need for the health care practitioner to develop their own systems approach to prescribing without creating undesirable drug interactions. A fundamental understanding of the clinical pharmacology of drug interactions and a framework for avoiding preventable drug interactions remains critically important. Thus we need to overlay technologic solutions on a base that is strong in basic principles of clinical pharmacology and drug interactions. Incorporation of up-to-date computerized databases is valuable, and frequent consultation with other members of the healthcare team, such as nurses and pharmacists, is essential.

Two more approaches to minimise ADRs are therapeutic drug monitoring and ADR monitoring. These are discussed in detail next two chapters.

CHAPTER SIXTEEN

Therapeutic Drug Monitoring (TDM)

Individualizing drug therapy is an important aspect of rational therapeutics. It involves choosing the appropriate drug(s) and dosage regimen(s) for each patient taking into account all the variables which can influence the ultimate drug effect(s). Drug effect, we know depends on tissue (receptor) sensitivity and amount of drug reaching the tissues. For some drugs, variation in amount of drug reaching to site of action is an important cause for variation in response. Individualizing drug dosage is important for drugs which have low therapeutic index. Dosage adjustment can be done by monitoring the effects clinically e.g. blood pressure for antihypertensives. But for many drugs, there is either is no readily available measure of effect or it is not sufficiently sensitive. For example clinical effects do not serve as good guidance when drugs are used prophylactically (e.g. anticonvulsants) or when drug effects develop slowly (e.g. antidepressants) or when drug effect cannot be differentiated from the complications of disease process (e.g. digoxin). For such drugs, measurement of plasma concentration is very useful. Plasma concentration indicates the dose required to achieve therapeutic levels for safe and effective outcome. Thus TDM involves measurement of drug concentration in body fluids and adjusting the dose in individual patients.

TDM is defined as "individualization of dosage by maintaining plasma or blood concentrations within a target range (therapeutic range/ therapeutic window). It is pragmatic manipulation of the dose of a drug using plasma concentration as a guide to optimize its efficacy, to avoid or identify toxicity and to detect or confirm poor compliance".

If the clinical effect can be readily measured (e.g. heart rate, blood pressure), it is obviously better to adjust the dose on the basis of response. Where this cannot be done, therapeutic drug monitoring is used in two major situations:

- Drugs used prophylactically to maintain the absence of a condition such as seizures, cardiac arrhythmias, depressive or manic episodes, asthma relapses or organ rejection.
- To avoid serious toxicity with narrow therapeutic range e.g. aminoglycoside antibiotics.

The characteristics of drugs which make them suitable for or make them require, therapeutic drug monitoring are:

- Marked pharmacokinetic variability.
- Concentration related therapeutic and adverse effects.
- Narrow therapeutic index.
- Defined therapeutic (target) concentration range.
- Desired therapeutic effect difficult to monitor.

The drugs for which TDM has been found to be useful are listed in Table16.1. For these drugs TDM is particularly indicated in the following clinical situations.

Table 16.1: Indications for TDM

Indication	*Drug/s*
Narrow therapeutic range	Lithium
Drugs with non-linear pharmacokinetics	Phenytoin
Drugs showing interindividual variation in biotransformation	Tricyclic antidepressants
Prophylactic use	Antiepileptics
To check toxicity	Salicylates
To check compliance	Antiepileptics
To check bioequivalence	Two or more brands of the same drug
To check drug interactions	Two or more drugs
To check effect of concomitant disease/ physiological conditions on drugs	Theophylline
Efficacy failure	Antiepileptics

The Important Steps in TDM are

Time of Sampling

The correct time of sampling is important. Drug concentrations vary over the dosing interval and with the duration of dosing in relation to achieving a steady state. This is unlike most physiological parameters such as serum creatinine or serum sodium which change relatively slowly. Generally, samples are collected after the steady state levels have been reached which takes approximately five half-lives. It is usually best to wait and assay at steady state unless there are concerns about toxicity. This does not apply to drugs such as amiodarone and perhexiline with very long half-lives and which can cause severe toxicity—steady state may take months to be reached and dose adjustments need to be made along the way. With all drugs, if a sample is taken before steady state is reached, allowance needs to be made for this in interpreting the concentration.

The least variable point in the dosing interval is the pre-dose or trough concentration. For drugs with short half-lives in relation to the dosing interval, samples should be collected pre-dose. For drugs with long half-lives such as phenytoin, phenobarbitone or amiodarone, samples collected at any point in the dosage interval can be satisfactory. For digoxin, any point after the distribution phase (after 6 hours post-dose) acceptable. It should also be remembered that therapeutic ranges have often been established using trough concentrations. If a patient is not responding to standard regimen and trough levels are within therapeutic range, before escalating the dose further, peak drug levels must be estimated to predict the maximum tolerated dose for that patient. Immediate sampling is recommended for in cases of suspected toxicity

Drug Estimation Methods

The sensitivity, specificity and reproducibility of the laboratory method is important. Most high-volume drug assays are now carried out by automated immunoassay methods which have these characteristics. However, a number continue to require manual assay by methods such as high performance liquid chromatography (HPLC) and gas liquid chromatography (GLC) (e.g. amiodarone, perhexiline). All methods if used correctly are acceptable. Participation in international quality control programmes will ensure laboratory validity. Recurring cost for HPLC is least of all. However it requires technical expertise. Usually, plasma or serum is used for drug assays, depending on the equipment used. However, with cyclosporin there are large shifts of drug between red cells and plasma with storage and temperature change so whole blood is assayed. Some blood collecting tubes, especially those containing a gel to separate cells and plasma, may not be suitable for all drugs due to drug adsorption by the gel or other components in the tube. All analytical methods estimate total drug (free + Protein bound) levels. Although it is the free drug which has direct access to the site of action In patients with normal plasma protein levels, total drug concentration correlates well with drug effects. However, sometimes it is necessary to estimate metabolites especially when the metabolite is active and the concentration is high (e.g. carbamazepine epoxide in children).

Interpretation of Plasma Concentration Data

The concentration measured must always be interpreted in the light of clinical response, the demographic and clinical status of individual patient, dosage regimen, concomitant drugs used. Ideally interpretation and advice should be there with each report. If the levels exceed 90% of therapeutic concentration, the dosage is halved. Dosage is further reduced by 50% if plasma levels exceed therapeutic concentrations at 4 half-life interval. If the first concentration is not too high, one can proceed with the same dose. With this procedure undue toxicity can be avoided.

Therapeutic concentrations are average values and individual patients will show satisfactory drug response at levels above and below the average values. Plasma concentration data must always be considered along with the patient's clinical response.

Dosage Adjustment

For drugs with linear kinetics increasing the dose leads to proportionate increase in plasma concentration and can be safely carried out. For drugs with nonlinear pharmacokinetics, relatively small increase in dosage can result in disproportionately large increase in plasma concentrations (e.g. phenytoin) for such a drug it is advisable to use a nomogram.

Nomograms are also available for dosage adjustment in renal insufficiency (e.g. aminoglycosides, antiarrhythmics).

A list of drugs for which therapeutic drug monitoring is commonly used is shown in table 16.2 with the target or therapeutic ranges. The ranges used are in most cases derived from observation of therapeutic and adverse effects in small groups of patients. Therefore, when applied to a wider population of patients, there will be individuals who achieve adequate effects at lower concentrations or experience adverse events within the 'therapeutic range'.

Table 16.2: Drugs and therapeutic range

Drug	***Time to steady state***	***Therapeutic range mg/L***
Digoxin	7 days	0.5 - 2.1
Amiodarone	1 month	1.0 - 2.5
Lignocaine	12 hours	2.0 - 5.0
Quinidine	24 hours	2.0 - 5.0
Mexilitine	2 days	0.5 - 2.5
Salicylate	2-5 days	150 - 300
Perhexiline		0.15 - 0.6
Theophylline	36 hours	10 - 20
Phenytoin	>2 weeks	10 - 20
Carbamazepine	2 weeks	5.0 - 12
Sodium valproate	40 hours	50 - 100
Phenobarbitone	2 weeks	15 - 40

Contd.

Contd.

Gentamicin, tobramycin, netilmicin	8 hours	trough 1-2; peak 5-10
Amikacin	8 hours	trough 3-5; peak 20-30
Lithium	3 days	0.6 - 1.2

The usual procedure followed for TDM is as given in figure 16.1.

Identify the clinical condition requiring TDM

↓

Collect sample at appropriate time

↓

Drug levels estimation using appropriate method

↓

Interpretation of result taking into account clinical response

Dosage adjustment ⇄ Effect

Repeat TDM to confirm achievement of target levels.

Fig.16.1: TDM procedure at a glance

With this background information let us now consider the important aspects of therapeutic drug monitoring of some of the drugs as related to ADRs.

Antiepileptic Drugs (AED)

Most antiepileptic drugs have a narrow margin of safety and there is considerable interindividual variation in pharmacokinetics, dosage requirement and response obtained.

Phenytoin

Measurement of plasma levels, commuting with effect, and adjusting the dose as per requirement is very important and rewarding for phenytoin. Phenytoin has a narrow margin of safety. Levels below l0 µg/ml do not give good seizure control and those above 20 µg/ml are associated with toxicity. However, do not consider plasma levels in isolation. It is seen that about 20% patients achieve good seizure control despite phenytoin levels below 10μg/ml on the other hand 3-5% patients are well controlled only with levels above 20 μg/ml and show no sign of toxicity. Patient compliance is a very important variable in AED treatment. When a patient shows subtherapeutic levels despite standard doses, compliance must be checked before increasing the dose. In majority of the patients receiving 300 mg phenytoin per day levels below 5 μg/ml were found to be simply due to non compliance. Patient counseling, simpler drug and dosage regimens, and recording intake helps to control seizures effectively in many patients.

Phenytoin has nonlinear kinetics and dose increments result in proportionately large increases in plasma concentrations leading to toxicity. Hence, it is necessary to use a nomogram for calculating dose requirement. Nomograms have been prepared using data from Western population. These can safely be used this for Indian population also.

One of the limitations of phenytoin tablets and capsules available in India is their dosage strength, all are of 100 mg strength (and syrup is 125 mg/5ml). On account of the nonlinear kinetics, dose increments of 100 mg can lead to toxic levels in some patients. It is observed that nearly 20% of the patients need dose increments of only 25 or 50 mg to achieve desired therapeutic concentrations. Appropriate dosage adjustment and achieving therapeutic concentration results in over 70% of patients getting good seizure control.

Carbamazepine

Therapeutic range of carbamazepine is 4-12 μg/ml. Plasma samples should be collected after steady state levels are reached. Some reduction in plasma concentration thereafter is to be expected on account of autoinduction. In adults, fluctuations in carbamazepine plasma levels between dosing intervals are not large and blood sample can be collected at trough or peak time. In children due to short half-life and specially with liquid formulations which can be rapidly absorbed, the difference between peak and trough levels can be substantial, requiring measurement of both levels depending on indication. Drug monitoring is most useful in deciding the extent to which dose can be increased in patients who are not responding to standard dose in spite of good compliance.

Phenobarbitone

Therapeutic range for phenobarbitone is 10 - 40 µg/ml and monitoring is mainly useful for deciding maximum increase in dose (side effect of drowsiness experienced by the patient is most important limiting factor).

Sodium Valproate

For sodium valproate, TDM is less critical as the correlation between effect and plasma level is not so good. However, TDM helps to confirm compliance and is useful in special situations like multiple drug therapy.

Antiarrhythmic Drugs

The primary objective of therapeutic drug monitoring in a patient with cardiac arrhythmia is to achieve an effective and well tolerated serum drug concentration as readily as possible and to maintain this concentration for as long as required without producing any adverse drug reactions. In most situations for most drugs, serum concentration after equilibrium strongly correlates with their antiarrhythmic effect as well as adverse effects of the drug(s). For checking efficacy, trough levels, are valuable while peak levels throw more light if drug toxicity is in question. One approach for optimizing-individualized antiarrhythmics drug therapy which is given in figure 16.2.

There are two basic approaches to select the first dose. First and the more commonly used one is to start with a loading dose and go on reducing till the target concentration is achieved. Second approach is to start, with the lowest dose and go on increasing till the target

Initiation or loading or maintenance dose

↓

Assessment of efficacy by programmed electrical pacing and EGG

↓

Effectiveness

↓

Obtaining serum drug concentration (trough level) (referred to as "Target" Concentration for that patient

↓

Maintaining on long term therapy (By obtaining periodic serum concentration)

↓

Keeping though concentration always more than target Concentration.

Fig. 16.2: Individualization of antiarrhythmics drug therapy

level is achieved, this approach is used for relatively more, toxic drugs like classic agents and amiodarone. Recently, a nomogram has also been made available to choose an initial dose of an antiarrhythmics agent for efficacy testing based on drug pharmacokinetics in healthy patients and in patients with organ dysfunction. These approaches for TDM are not currently being practiced in India because of lack of resources in the field. In spite of its great usefulness, therapeutic monitoring for arrhythmic drugs is not without its limitations. Some of the important limitations are as follows:

1. Antiarrhythmics effect of the drug depends not only on plasma drug level but also on the type of arrhythmia e.g. procainamide can control a trial arrhythmias at much, lower concentration than recurrent ventricular tachycardia. The abolition of reentrant arrhythmia is a dynamic process that requires a critical balance of refractoriness and conduction velocity. Thus, a drug may prevent the reentrant mechanism at low concentration but at a higher concentration the resultant elect physiological effects may again allow reentry.
2. Disopyramide shows anticholinergic effects and mexiletine produces neurotoxicity at concentrations

above 5μg/ml and 2μg/ml respectively. On the other hand, some toxicity has little or no correlation with plasma levels e.g. proarrhythmic effect (torsades de pointes) occurs at low to therapeutic concentrations of quinidine.

3. The target concentrations for long term maintenance therapy are based on the concentrations effective in suppressing arrhythmias induced by electrical programmed stimulation. However, CAST-trial has shown that such suppression may not correlate with the long term effectiveness of a drug.
4. There is a plethora of new antiarrhythmics agents which have been recently released or are in clinical trials. However, scarce data exists regarding their effective concentrations and concentration effect relations.

Digitalis

The clinical usefulness of serum digitalis levels has been the subject of considerable controversy and debate. Although there is reasonable correlation between serum levels and inotropic effect, the same does not necessarily exist for electrophysiological effects. The inotropic response is altered by other interventions such as bed rest, oxygen, sedation, diuretics, or reduction of blood pressure. The status of autonomic nervous system, presence of disease, electrolyte disturbances and other host factors influence the electrophysiological effects.

Serum levels between 0.8 and 2 mg/ml for digoxin and between 15 and 25 mg/ml for digitoxin are usually associated with a satisfactory inotropic response and a low risk of toxicity. In supraventricular arrhythmias however, higher plasma levels (2-4 mg/ml of digoxin) may be needed to control the ventricular rate. These values related to steady state conditions and very high peak concentrations achieved during intravenous loading doses can be safe.

The risk of toxicity increases with levels higher than those mentioned above, but there is considerable overlap. In one study 25% of patients with digitalis toxicity had levels in the therapeutic range and 15% without toxicity had levels beyond the range.

A serum digoxin level below 2ng/ml does not necessarily avoid noncardiac symptoms of toxicity. Thus digitalis toxicity is and will undoubtedly remain a clinical diagnosis. Serum level data only gives additional information.

But there are instances where serum level is clearly beneficial e.g. when clinical response is appropriate for prescribed dose serum levels help in the question of noncompliance, low bioavailability (fatty diet decreases absorption), faulty or altered metabolism. Serum levels data is invaluable in deciding dosages in patients with pharmacokinetic drug interactions. Some old patients need extremely large doses, poor absorption being the probable reason.

Lithium

Lithium is an important drug for the treatment of acute mania and for long term preventive treatment of bipolar manic depressive disorders. However it has a narrow margin of safety and there is considerable interindividual variation. Lithium is excreted, through the kidney and the variation in renal clearance contributes significantly to the variation in the dose requirement. Slow disintegration of lithium preparations and diarrhea can reduce absorption, while sodium poor diet, slimming diet, concomitant treatment with diuretics enhance elimination. Thus lithium intoxication occur intercurrently during unchanged treatment. Monitoring plasma lithium level helps to avoid it and tailor make lithium dose to individual patient requirement. Lithium is given in divided doses of 1200-1800 mg per day for acute mania (to give levels of 0.8-1.0 meq/L) and maintenance dose of 900-1200 mg (to give levels of 0.6-1.0 meq/L). The sample for therapeutic drug monitoring should be collected at steady state i.e. one week after the last lithium dose with an accuracy of ±30 min. The biological half life of lithium is longer during night time and morning concentrations will be considerably higher than the corresponding evening sample. It is therefore recommended that blood sample collection time should be standardized to morning time. Many patient on long term therapy do well at levels between 0.6 and 0.8 meq/L and many even between 0.4-0.6 meq/L. As serum levels rises above 1.5 meq/L the likelihood of lithium intoxication increases.

The most common adverse reactions are: neurological intoxication, hypothyroidism and nephrotoxicity. Rarely a sensitive patient will become clinically toxic at therapeutic levels if slow release form is given twelve hourly. Post dose value is higher by 30% than if the same dose is given as regular tablets in split dose. Levels obtained two hours after the dose give high values and should not form basis for dose reduction. Drug interactions with most NSAIDs except aspirin and sulindac reduces renal clearance and increase lithium levels.

Therapeutic drug monitoring is indispensable in lithium therapy. It is also essential that patients and relatives are trained to supervise treatment. In the elderly, longer half life and increased sensitivity to side effects are important considerations and the starting dose should be low. As the elimination half life increases, longer time will be required to reach steady state. After discontinuation, serum levels fall more slowly and resolution of toxicity and side effects may be delayed. In pregnancy dose should be closely watched. Lithium is a teratogen affecting cardiovascular system. Fetal echocardiography may be a useful test for detecting major cardiovascular malformations.

One of the methods of determining the lithium dose is to administer a single test dose of 600 mg and then measure the serum levels 24 hours later. According to the level at that time, one can make a prediction about the daily need to provide serum concentration between 0.6–1.2 meq/L. This procedure may be particularly useful in patients with mild renal impairment or any other condition that might lead to unpredictable serum lithium concentrations. This method has been further modified with a change in test dose to 900 mg and formulation of a nomogram now for predicting daily dose based on serum levies at twenty four hours.

It should be adequate to measure serum level of lithium weekly during the first four weeks of treatment and less often (every four to six weeks) thereafter. The trend towards lower dosage and lower serum concentrations may decrease side effects and complications of treatment. However, patients who do not respond should be treated, with the highest doses that are tolerable.

Tricyclic Antidepressants

There, is considerable (over ten fold) variation in plasma levels achieved in different patients receiving same dose of tricyclic antidepressant and there is thus a corresponding variation in the dose required. This variability seems to be genetically determined and stems from differences in rates of metabolism, further modified by age, disease state and interactions. For assessment of severity of depressive illness and response to treatment the clinician has to rely on his clinical observations and patient's report of his subjective symptoms. Rating scales help to quantitate response. However recovery from depression with drug treatment is a slow and gradual process and titration of dosage on the basis of clinical effect is inevitably delayed until the clinician is able to judge response with certainty. With most tricyclic antidepressants steady state levels develop by a week suggesting that time could be saved by plasma level measurement and dosage adjustment early in treatment. Side effects develop earlier in treatment but are of little use for titration of dosage because they mimic symptoms of depression(tiredness, dry mouth, constipation) and anxiety (palpitation, sweating, dizziness). Plasma levels may help to achieve a minimal effective dose more quickly and more reliably. However, It must he remembered that the relationship between plasma concentration and effect is not so clear cut and is not Linear

Concentration Effect Relationship

There are three possible relationships of plasma level and efficacy:

1. Inverted U Shaped relationship: It was noted for nortryptyline trial drug loses its efficacy at high plasma levels. Patients with plasma levels above 180 ng/ml showed improvement in response when the levels were reduced. While the patients with levels below 50ng/ml did not respond.
2. No relationship: A number of studies of amitriptyline were unable to demonstrate clearly upper and lower limit of therapeutic window.
3. Threshold level for improvement: With imipramine, therapeutic response is seen in less (33%) patients with level below 180 ng/ml (probably placebo response) while 70% of those with levels above 240 ng/ml responded. The range is not absolute and in some studies value different from these have been noted.

The therapeutic drug monitoring of tricyclic antidepressants is indicated in elderly, those with cardiac illness, patients developing disturbing subjective side effect with modest dosage and patients who do not respond to treatment with standard dosages.

Antipsychotic Drugs

It is noted that patients taking comparable doses of antipsychotic manifest widely varying plasma levels. Most drugs show increasing side effects as plasma level increase and with some drugs there is a paradoxical loss of efficacy with high plasma levels.

At this time however antipsychotic plasma levels are not feasible for clinical use. Methods for measuring plasma levels remain technically complex and drugs e.g. chlorpromazine have many metabolites which complicates interpretation of data.

Antibiotics

Aminoglycosides: The aminoglycosides antibiotics are potent bactericidal agents commonly used to treat severe gram negative infections. However, use of these agents is limited by their low therapeutic Indices and marked inter and intra individual pharmacokinetic variations especially in patients with imparted renal functions. Determination of plasma drug concentration therefore helps in adequate dosage adjustment. Since aminoglycosides have short half-fives, both peak (sample collected 30 minutes after a 30 minute infusion) and trough (sample collected just prior to the next infusion) should be obtained. Optimal peak levels ensure adequacy of antimicrobial activity whereas trough levels help in detecting drug accumulation (toxicity).

What Information is Required for Interpretation?

Drug concentrations need to be interpreted in the context of the individual patient without rigid adherence to a therapeutic range. The basic information about the sample and the patient required for adequate interpretation of a drug concentration is shown in Table 16.3. Besides this, a good knowledge of the disposition of the drug is needed. There are two important factors which can make interpretation of a result difficult in some cases. These are changes in protein binding and active metabolites.

Table 16.3: Information required to interpret TDM results

- Time of sample in relation to last dose
- Duration of treatment with the current dose
- Dosing schedule
- Age, gender
- Other drug therapy
- Relevant disease states
- Reason for request e.g. lack of effect, routine monitoring, suspected toxicity

Special Issues

Assays are done using plasma or blood and thus measure bound and unbound drug, whereas it is the unbound drug that interacts with the receptor to produce a response. If binding is changed by disease states, displacement by another drug or non-linearity in protein binding, the interpretation of total plasma or blood drug concentrations must be modified. For example, the therapeutic range for phenytoin based on total drug concentration is 10-20 mg/L which corresponds to an unbound drug concentration of 1-2 mg/L (fraction unbound, f_u is normally 0.1). If f_u is increased to 0.2, as, for example, in renal disease, the target unbound concentration is still 1-2 mg/L, but the therapeutic range for total drug is 5-10 mg/L. Unless this is realised, inappropriate dose adjustments may be made, resulting in toxicity. Sodium valproate and salicylate show non-linear binding in the therapeutic range making interpretation of total drug concentrations difficult.

Active Metabolites

Metabolites which may not be measured can contribute to the therapeutic response. Examples include carbamazepine (carbamazepine-10,11-epoxide), and procainamide (N-acetylprocainamide). Theophylline in neonates (but not in adults) is converted to caffeine, so the therapeutic range for theophylline in neonatal apnoea is 6-12 mg/L (allowing for the contribution of caffeine), whereas it is 10-20 mg/L for obstructive airways disease in adults. The therapeutic ranges for imipramine and amitriptyline are based on the combined concentrations of parent drug and active metabolite (desipramine and nortriptyline respectively). Finally, primidone treatment is monitored by measuring the concentration of the active metabolite phenobarbitone, but primidone itself and another metabolite, phenylethylmalonamide, are also active.

Is TDM Cost-effective?

Therapeutic drug monitoring is now so taken for granted that the difficulties in managing some drugs without it are forgotten. While the digoxin therapeutic range is somewhat 'loose', the advent of monitoring resulted in a far greater appreciation of the toxicity of digoxin and of the need for rational dosing. Similarly, theophylline, while now falling out of favour for other reasons, was rescued from oblivion when the advent of therapeutic drug monitoring in the 1970s allowed its use largely without the serious toxicity previously associated with it. The use of any of the drugs in Table 16.2 without monitoring would be difficult and often dangerous. Emphasis should be placed not so much on whether monitoring is necessary as on how to use it in the most cost-effective and clinically effective manner possible.

CHAPTER SEVENTEEN

ADR Monitoring

It took many decades before the deleterious effects of aspirin on the gastrointestinal tract became apparent and almost as long before it was recognised that the protracted abuse of phenacetin could produce renal papillary necrosis; 35 years elapsed before it became clear that amidopyrine could cause agranulocytosis; and several years before the association of phocomelia with thalidomide became obvious. Hence, systematic collection of information on adverse drug is essential to provide much needed information regarding patients at risk, drug interactions and adverse reactions to new drugs not detected in studies conducted before marketing of the drug.

Health professionals are in the best position to report on suspected ADRs observed in their every day patient care. All healthcare providers (physicians, pharmacists, nurses, dentists and others) should report ADRs as part of their professional responsibility, even if they are doubtful about the precise relationship with the given medication. You can reduce the suffering and save thousands of patients lives by doing this. ADR monitoring is to help ensure that patients obtain safe and efficacious products. The results of ADR monitoring have also a very important educational value.

Several methods used for collection of information on adverse reactions to drugs have been reported in literature. The main methods are as follows:

Premarketing Clinical Trials

Before marketing of drug, animal studies and human trials (Phase I, II and III) are done to detect ADRs. Animal studies include acute, subacute, chronic toxicity studies and specialized toxicity studies. But, it has been proved again and again that tests in animals are insufficient to predict human safety. Clinical trial done in humans to look for ADRs, but number of patients is limited and there trials detect ADR with an incidence of 1:200 only. The declared purpose of 'pre-marketing' clinical trials is to discover:

- If a drug works and how well.
- If it has any harmful effects.
- If there is potential harm how serious is it and how does it weigh against the benefits.

There are concerns about these premarketing studies because of two reasons:

1. Before marketing drugs are evaluated for toxicity in animals. These studies produce an overall picture of toxicology of the drug and indicate organs which are at highest risk of damage. However, it is difficult to draw direct parallels between toxicity in animal models and potential risks to man.
2. After animal toxicity studies drug undergoes clinical trials in humans. For a new drug pre-marketing clinical trials are generally carried out in less than 3000 patients. Type A reactions can thus be identified. Subgroups at particular risks are occasionally identified. However, type B reactions with incidence of 1:1000 are generally missed.

By the time of licensing, exposure of less than 5000 human subjects to a drug allows only the more common ADR to be detected. At least 30,000 people need to be treated with a drug to be sure that you do not miss at least one patient with an ADR which has an incidence of 1 in 10,000 exposed individuals. Patients used in clinical trials are selected and limited in number, the conditions of use differ from those in clinical practice and the duration of trials is limited. Even detected events will be incompletely described and understood, since they are too few. Susceptible population like elderly are unlikely to be included in these studies and effects of intercurrent disease or medication are poor. Hence, a drug that is tested in a few thousand people may have an excellent safety profile in those few thousand patients. However, within a short time after entering the market, the drug may be administered to several million patients. That means that for drugs that cause rare toxicity, their toxicity can only be detected after, not before marketing.

So, the safety profile for new drugs that come on the market is never totally defined because new drugs are studied only in relatively small and homogenous patient populations. The complete safety profile of a new drug will be defined only after it has been approved and is in use on the market.

Clinical trials generally do tell a good deal about how well a drug works for a defined disease and what potential harm it may cause. However they provide no information for larger populations with different characteristics from the trial group-age, gender, state of health, ethnic origin and so on.

Therefore, for many medicines, and particularly new, complex products, safety monitoring does not stop at the manufacturing stage; it must be followed by careful patient monitoring and by further scientific data collection. This aspect of drug monitoring is called post-marketing.

Post-marketing Methods

In these methods ADRs are observed epidemiologically under conditions of normal use in the community. Thus, post-marketing surveillance is important to permit detection of less common, but sometimes very serious ADRs. Therefore health professionals worldwide should report on ADRs as it can save lives of their patients and others. The various methods used are:

Case Reports: This has the advantage of speed and sensitivity, however the reports need to be validated.

Case reports have been the first means by which some of the type B reactions have been identified e.g. Practolol induced dermatitis and keratoconjunctivitis, benoxaprofen induced photosensitivity which is dose related.

Cohort Studies: Cohort of patients receiving a drug under investigation are prospectively studied and compared with control population. The cohort studies are excellent methods of quantifying ADRs e.g. Royal College of General Practitioner's oral contraceptive study. The contraceptive study quantified the risk of cardiovascular diseases and excess mortality due to oral contraceptives. However cohort studies are expensive and slow and do not necessarily, prove causal link.

Prescription Event Monitoring: Patients who have received specific drugs are identified from prescription (in UK prescription pricing authority). The general practitioner is then asked to report any adverse event detected. The method has the advantage of enhancing detection of new adverse reactions and incidence of event can be calculated. Prescription event monitoring has identified deafness associated with enalapril.

Case Control Studies (Retrospective): In this Prospective method patients who have the identified disease are matched with a control group who have similar potentially confounding factors but who do not have the disease. The drug histories are then compared. The association between aspirin and Reye's syndrome was confirmed using this method and resulted in recommending removal of the pediatric formulation of aspirin from the market.

Spontaneous Reporting-Yellow Card System: Spontaneous reporting of ADRs to a central body was started in UK in 1964. However it is estimated that out of even serious and fatal ADRs, only 10% are reported so there is gross underreporting. Reporting may be biased and limited to serious ADRs. Advantages of this system are that numbers are large, personal details are kept confidential and early alerts are available. The yellow card system identified the risk of urticaria and confirmed the occurrence of cough due to captopril and enalapril. It is recommended that a physician for newer drugs a physician must report all suspected ADRs and for established drugs, he should report all serious suspected ADRs. Advantages of this system is that it acts as early alerting system.

Record Linkage: The health records of a defined population are correlated with data on the use of drugs. This technique is not very sensitive compared to other methods but can generate hypotheses for further investigation.

Advantages include:

1. Large sample size.
2. No recall bias.
3. Records are confidential.

Disadvantages are:

1. Skewed population.
2. All information not recorded.
3. Risk factors not included.

Phase-IV Clinical Studies (Post-marketing Surveillance): Post-marketing surveillance (PMS) is an regulatory requirement and done for all the drugs after marketing. This surveillance provides information of long term safety of drug, safety in extremes of ages, safety in special population e.g. pregnant and lactating females. Severe ADRs may lead to withdrawal of drugs. In India it is now mandatory to submit results of postmarketing surveillance within 2 years of marketing the drug. Sometimes after this surveillance warnings on ADRs are inserted on labels of drugs.

This monitoring can be done as regional or national level. Other way to monitor is to monitor disease, rather than drugs, especially in case of Type B bizarre ADRs, that will help in identifying many serious adverse effects in different subspecialities of medicine and surgery e.g. carcinoma in young females showed unusual clear cell carcinoma like histopathological features, only in these mothers who received stilboestrol during pregnancy, similarly biopsy revealed pseudomembranous colitis in those treated with tetracycline lead to the path of drugs induced adverse effect in the gastroenterology department, while ophthalmic department could observe a different kind of dry eye in those treated with controlled care studies. Thus orientation and participation of physicians can help identifying the new drugs reaction, as well as minimizing the adverse effect of dugs through regularly updating their own knowledge.

WHO promotes drug safety through its International Drug Monitoring Programme, which began to operate in 1968. Initially a pilot project in 10 countries with established national reporting systems for ADRs, the network has expanded significantly as more countries worldwide develop national pharmacovigilance centers for the recording of ADRs. Currently, 86 countries participate in the programme.

The Uppsala Monitoring Centre (UMC, WHO), Sweden is maintaining the international database of adverse drug reaction (ADR) reports received from several National Centers. In September 2005, the database had 3.5 million adverse drug reaction reports and 78 countries were participating in this programme. Vigibase online (web based) system is used for submission of ADR reports. Although, India is participating in this programme, its contribution to UMC database is very little. This is essentially due to the absence of a vibrant ADR monitoring system and also the lack of a reporting culture among health care workers.

The most important task of the Drug Monitoring Programme is to identify 'signals' of drug safety problems as early as possible. A signal is defined by WHO as 'reported information on a possible causal relationship between an adverse event and a drug' which has not been previously detected.

Reported cases of ADRs are forwarded from national pharmacovigilance centers to the WHO Collaborating Centre for International Drug Monitoring in Uppsala, Sweden. The case reports are stored in the ADR data base. Over 3.1 million case records are maintained in the data base, the most comprehensive source of international ADR information.

In addition, WHO also:

- Has established a system for regular exchange of information between Member States on the safety and efficacy of pharmaceutical products, using a network of designated national information officers.
- Ensures the prompt transmission to national health authorities of new information on serious adverse effects of pharmaceutical products.
- Devises and disseminates guidelines to set up national drugs monitoring centers.
- Trains doctors and drug safety monitoring experts across the globe on new and complex medicines (i.e. antiretrovirals).
- Works with countries to strengthen drug regulatory authorities and establish reporting systems for ADRs.
- Facilitates contacts between major stakeholders (regulatory authorities, police, customs officials, etc.) to combat counterfeit medicines at a national, regional and global level.

A well-organized drug safety management "pharmacovigilance" service is a prerequisite for the early detection of the risks of drugs, prevention of adverse drug reactions and aiding health professionals and patients to make the best benefit/risk assessment for safe and effective pharmacotherapy. WHO defines pharmacovigilance as "the science and activities relating to the detection, assessment, understanding and prevention of ADRs or any other, medicine-related problem". Pharmacovigilance plays a major role in pharmacotherapy decision-making, be it individual, regional, national or international.

Medicine induced morbidity and mortality can be substantially reduced through an integrated strategy for drug safety monitoring which includes:

- Establishment of the national pharmacovigilance service.
- Education and training of health care professionals on benefit/risk assessment and rational use of drugs.
- Behaviour change amongst patients and healthcare workers to decrease unnecessary and irrational use of drugs.

Special Need for ADR Monitoring in India

Due to huge population, unorganized health sector, use of alternative medicine there is an urgent need for monitoring ADRs in India.

a. *Population variation:* It is known that there is variation in ADRs between different countries on account of variation in genetic, environmental, dietary factors and disease patterns and drug used. The incidence of drug induced hepatotoxicity is low in India compared to Western data. The common drugs incriminated were antitubercular drugs as opposed to halothane reported to be the commonest in the Danish registry.

b. *Nutritional status:* In India, in rural areas, 45-70% of population is iron deficient, over 50% of children are malnourished which may affect incidence of ADR.

c. *Paucity of data:* There are very few functioning centers in India. Adequate information is not available even on adverse reactions to old drugs. There is paucity of data on ADR in specialised populations like pregnant, women and children.

d. *Peculiarities of drug usage in India:* Due to the increased prevalence of certain diseases in this country certain drugs are used in a population where they are not recommended e.g. Ciprofloxacin in children.

e. *Traditional system of medicine:* Many patients tend to use modern drugs along with traditional remedies. Interactions that can result could lead to adverse reaction and loss of efficacy. Traditional drugs are considered safe but may not necessarily be safe.

Organization of ADR Monitoring System in India

Appreciating the importance and benefits of pharmacovigilance, Central Drugs Standard Control Organization (CDSCO), Ministry of Health and Family Welfare, Govt. of India launched the National Pharmacovigilance Programme (NPP) in November, 2004. It is largely based on the recommendations made in the WHO document titled "Safety Monitoring of Medicinal Products - Guidelines for Setting Up and Running a Pharmacovigilance Centre".

The immediate aim of NPP is to foster the culture of ADR notification by health care workers. Subsequently, it seeks to generate broad based ADR data on the Indian population and share this with UMC, WHO database. This would ensure optimum safety of drug products in the Indian market.

Under this programme, the whole country is divided into zones and regions for operational efficiency. CDSCO, New Delhi is at the top of the hierarchy followed by two zonal pharmacovigilance centers viz, Seth GS Medical College, Mumbai and AIIMS, New Delhi. There are 5 regional pharmacovigilance centers located at Kolkata *(IPGMR-SSKM Hospitals)*, Mumbai *(TN Medical College and BYL Nair Charitable Hospital)*, Nagpur *(Indira Gandhi Medical College)*, New Delhi *(Lady Hardinge Medical College)* and Pondicherry *(JIPMER)*. Twenty eight peripheral centers, spread country-wide, are attached to their nearest peripheral centers. ADR reports can be sent only by healthcare workers (doctors including dentists, nurses, pharmacists) to any one of the nearest pharmacovigilance centre. The full list of centers is available at CDSCO web site (www.cdsco.nic.in). ADR reports sent by lay public are not acceptable. Data received at the peripheral centers are forwarded to the respective regional centers which will carry out the causality analysis. This information will be forwarded to the zonal centers. From there the data will be forwarded to the CDSCO and UMC database. The ADR form for reporting ADRs in India is given in the last chapter (Table 19.11).

The functioning of NPP is to be periodically reviewed by the National Pharmacovigilance Advisory Committee" — a 16-member committee appointed by the Govt. of India. The committee will also evaluate the pharmacovigilance data received from various centers and recommend possible regulatory measures.

ADR monitoring programmes are not new to India. In 1982, five centers were established by Drug Controller General of India for nationwide monitoring of ADR. In 1987, ICMR had collected about 58,000 ADR cases through its multi-institutional study but they all stopped functioning after few years due to several reasons such as insufficient funds, lack of enthusiasm etc. The present programme may be successful since this has been structured taking into consideration the past deficiencies. Three interactive workshops were conducted by CDSCO/WHO for training the participants of the programme. Further, the World Bank has committed to provide US $1,00,000 for this project. The success of this programme depends on the continuous active support by CDSCO and the dedicated work of the pharmacovigilance centers.

A national strategy should be developed that ensures that pharmacovigilance services at all levels adhere to national and international regulations and standards. This can be achieved by following:

- National regulations and guidelines for drug monitoring should be approved and implemented in the country.
- Guidelines on ADR control and reporting and case-report forms should be available to all healthcare professionals.
- Make contact with the health authorities and with local, regional or national institutions and groups, working in clinical medicine, pharmacology and toxicology outlining the importance of pharmacovigilance and its purposes.
- Produce printed materials to inform health professionals about definitions, aims and methods of the pharmacovigilance.
- An adequate number of trained staff should be available in hospitals or regions in accordance with their needs.
- Organize meetings in hospitals, academia and professional associations, explaining the principles and demands of pharmacovigilance and the importance of reporting.

- Set up a Pharmacovigilance Centre(s) and maintain its activities.

One example to overcome problem of ADRs in postmarketing surveillance can be taken from policies of Japanese health ministry. In their setup, the pharmaceutical industry is required to provide their product to a limited number of medical institutions for a period of three months following launch of a product and conduct focused post marketing surveillance. After inspection of data of this surveillance, the manufacturer are then allowed to expand number of medical institutions. Limiting sales to few institutions and Collecting information in this way makes it easier to respond to ADRs of newly approved drugs.

Systematic collection of data on ADR as mentioned above provides information on incidence, establishes causality and may identify risk factors.

Reasoning for Poor ADR Monitoring

1. Doctors feel that they are trained to treat patients and not monitor ADRs.
2. Government has no effective machinery to monitor ADRs.
3. Patient communities can not report an ADR.
4. There is non law which makes it mandatory for physicians to report ADRs.
5. Premarketing studies are grossly inadequate to detect ADRs <1 in 100-10000 patients.
6. No guarantee of confidentiality of a reported ADR by a doctor.
7. Population is not educated about ADRs and interprets it as doctor's negligence.

Summary of points required to effectively deal with ADRs:

- Make sure that sufficient information is provided to consumers on the efficacy and safety of products as well as contraindications.
- Setup right channels for consumers to report ADRs and make those channels known.

- Organise communication campaigns to equip consumers with the ability to discern the quality of service they receive.
- Ensure that practitioners are appropriately qualified and registered.
- Encourage interaction between traditional and conventional practitioners.
- Provide insurance for non-conventional therapies and products whose evidence base is sound.
- Health system structure and processes would help promote better quality and safety.
- Development of quality standards and treatment guidelines to ensure uniformity within a particular health system.

CHAPTER EIGHTEEN

ADRs and CPA (Consumer Protection Act)

In March, 2006 a US-based Indian doctor has claimed damages to the tune of over Rs 77 crore from a private clinic and three Kolkata-based doctors for the death of his wife allegedly caused due to "wrong" treatment given to her in May last year.

The doctor in a complaint filed before the National Consumer Disputes Redressal Commission (NCDRC) here recently, said, the doctors were liable to pay the damages and also sought to initiate appropriate action against the doctors responsible for prescribing "wrong" treatment to his wife.

According to the complaint, the damages were claimed taking into account her annual salary of $ 30,000, expenses on treatment in India and traveling including from USA and the mental agony caused to the complainant. The compensation demanded includes special damages of Rs 10 crore from the doctor who initially examined her and Rs 10 crore from two other doctors who treated her subsequently when shifted to a private clinic. He had named 16 other doctors as respondents in his plea and sought appropriate action against them for their alleged role in treating his wife.

This in one of the few cases doctors are facing routinely. The medical treatment is presently under the preview of CPA. This happened after the honorable Supreme Court's judgment in the landmark case in *Indian Medical Association Vs V.P. Shantha and Others* in 1995.

As a result of this judgment, medical profession has been brought under the section 2(1) (o) of CPA, 1986 and also, it has included the following categories of doctors/hospitals under this section:

1. All medical/dental practitioners doing independent medical/dental practice unless rendering only free service.
2. Private hospitals charging all patients.
3. All hospitals having free as well as paying patients and all the paying and free category patients receiving treatment in such hospitals.
4. Medical/dental practitioners and hospitals paid by an insurance firm for the treatment of a client or an employment for that of an employee.

It exempts only those hospitals and the medical / dental practitioners of such hospitals which offer free service to all patients.

As a result of this judgment, virtually all private and government hospitals and the doctors employed by them and the independent medical/dental practitioners except primary health centers, birth control measures, anti malaria drive and other such welfare activities can be sued under the CPA.

On the meaning of the word "service" in relation to medical profession, the Supreme Court in *Indian Medical Association v. V.P. Shantha and Ors.* came to the following conclusions:

- Service rendered to a patient by a medical practitioner (except) where the doctor rendered service free of charge to every patient or under a contract of personal service), by way consultation, diagnosis and treatment, both medicinal and surgical, would fall within the ambit of 'service' as defined in section 2(1) (o) of the Act.
- The expression 'contract of personal service' in section 2(1) (o) of the Act cannot be confined to contracts for employment of domestic servants only and the said expression would include the employment of a medical officer for the purpose of rendering medical service to the employer. The

service rendered by a medical officer to his employer under the contract of employment would be outside the purview of 'service' as defined in section 2(1) (o) of the Act.

- Service render at a Government hospital/health centre/dispensary or at non-government hospital/ nursing home where no charge whatsoever is made from any person availing the service and all patients (rich and poor) are given free service- is outside the purview of the expression "service" as defined in section 2(1) (o) of the Act. The payment of a token amount for registration purpose only at the hospital/ nursing home would not alter the position.
- Service rendered at a non-government hospital/ nursing home where charges are required to be paid by the person availing such services falls within the purview of the expression 'service' as defined in section 2(1) (o) of the Act.
- Service rendered at Government hospital/Health centre/ Dispensary or at a non-government Nursing home where charges are required to be paid by persons who are in a position to pay and persons who cannot afford to pay are rendered service free of charge would fall within the ambit of the expression 'service' as defined in section 2(1) (o) of the Act irrespective of the fact that the service is rendered free of charge to persons who are not in a position to pay for such services. Free service, by such doctors and hospitals would also be 'service' and the recipient a 'consumer' under the Act.
- Service rendered by a medical or hospital/nursing home cannot be regarded as service rendered free of charge, if the persons availing the service has taken an insurance policy for medical care where under the policy charges for consultation diagnosis and medical treatment are borne by the insurance company and such service would fall within the ambit of 'service' as defined in section 2(1) (o) of the Act.
- Similarly, where as a part of the conditions of service, the employer bears the expenses of medical treatment of an employee and his family member dependent

on him, the service rendered to such an employee and his family members by a medical practitioner or a hospital/nursing home would not be free of charge and would constitute 'service' under section 2(1) (o) of the Act.

CONSUMER DISPUTES REDRESSAL AGENCIES

Redressal Forums have been established as three different levels:

- "District Forum" by State Government. At least one in each district in certain cases on District Forum may cover 2 or more district, or there may be two or more District Forums in one District.
- "State Commission" by State Government.
- "National Commission" (National Consumer Disputes Redressal Commission) by Central Government.

DO'S AND DON'TS FOR DOCTORS

Don'ts for Doctors

- Don't prescribe without examining the patient, even if he is a close friend or relative (Telephone advice is an exception).
- It may not be reasonable for a doctor to assume what the patient is saying is truthful where what the patient/ attendant says is clearly contradicted by the symptoms.
- Don't prescribe a drug or indulge in a procedure of you cannot justify its indication.
- Don't prescribe a drug or indulge in a procedure of you cannot justify its indication.
- Don't prescribe/administer a drug which is banned, e.g. Analgin.
- Don't over-prescribe/administer too much of the drug, too large a dose, for too long.
- Don't under-prescribe: not prescribing the needed drug, dose is too small, length of treatment is too short.
- Don't prescribe multiple drugs. Such prescription may be due to inability to form a correct diagnosis

or other causes. Possibilities of drug interactions increase with polypharmacy.

- Don't write instructions on a separate slip. Don't allow substitutions.
- Don't adopt experimental method in treatment. If there is some rationale do it only after informed consent.
- Don't do anything beyond your level of competence. Competence is defined by your qualification, training and experience.

Do's for Doctors

- Mention your qualifications/training/experience/ designation on the prescription. Qualifications mean recognized degrees/diplomas as regulated by the Indian Medical Degrees Act, 1916 as amended from time to time. Mention of scholarships/membership/ awards which are no qualifications should be avoided.
- Always mention date and timing of the consultation.
- Mention age and sex of the patient. In a pediatric prescription weight of the patient must also be mentioned.
- Mention "diagnosis under review" until the diagnosis is finally settled.
- In complicated cases record precisely history of illness and substantial physical findings about the patient on your prescription.
- If the patient/attendants are erring on any count (history not reliable, refusing investigations, refusing admission) make a note of it or seek written refusal preferably in local language with proper witness.
- Mention the condition of patient in specific/objective terms. Avoid vague/non-specific terminology.
- Record history of drug allergy.
- Write names of drugs clearly. Use correct dosages (by revising knowledge periodically) and mention clearly method and interval of administration. Here one must use local or sign language. Do not forget writing precautions like Ast./ p.c./ a.c./ locally/ with milk/ h.s.etc. in local language.

- If a drug is a poison (e.g., certain local applications), warn in writing.
- Mention additional precautions, e.g., food, rest, avoidance of certain drugs, allergens, alcohol, smoking, etc., if indicated.
- Give instruction to the patient in comprehensible terms, making sure that the patient understands both the instruction and the importance of strictly adhering to them, e.g., while prescribing to potent anti-inflammatory drug, warn that if he experience any stomach trouble he should stop taking the drug and consult a doctor immediately.
- Mention likely side-effects, and action to be taken if they occur.
- Remember to advise in writing pathological tests/radiological tests at specified intervals for certain drugs which require such monitoring if such drugs are prescribed. Some examples are: Sodium Valporate, Carbamazepine, Gold Salts, Methotrexate and other Immuno-suppressives, Chloramphenicol, etc.
- Always advise the patient not to stop taking a drug suddenly which is required to be tapered before it is stopped. Remember major drug interactions.
- Specifically mention review, SOS/or follow-up schedule.
- Mention if patient/attendant are/is under effect of alcohol/drugs.
- In case a particular drug/equipment is not available, make a note.
- Prescribe with caution during pregnancy/lactation.
- Adjust doses in case of a child/elderly patient and in renal or hepatic disorders.
- In case of chronic ailments, mention treatment to be taken immediately in case of an emergency. For example, a patient on antiepileptic treatment should be advised to take an injection of diazepam when convulsions occur. In case of any deviation from standard care, mention reasons.
- Whenever referring a patient, provide him with a referring note.

In case of emergency/serious illness, ring up the concerned doctor in the patient's presence. Show your concern. Always keep with you and refer the latest edition of the standard text book of your branch of medicine. Always subscribe to at least one standard journal and participate in at least updates/ conferences every year.

- Medication to relieve pain especially in post-operative and cancer cases must be carried our carefully.
- Always obtain a legally valid consent before undertaking surgical/diagnostic procedure. Learn the difference between "informed persuasion" and "informed consent". The first is legally wrong, through at times it may be medically correct.
- While administering an injection/vaccination always check:
  - Name of the injection (a wrong injection may be given by mistake or oversight).
  - Expiry date.
  - Reconfirm the route of administration.
  - If it is to be diluted, check the dilution factor (1:2, 1:4 etc.).
  - Rate of administration (fast, slow, in drip, etc.).
  - Site of infection, e.g. antero-lateral, thigh, if age 1 year, gluteal region, deltoid, etc.
  - That a disposable syringe and needle are used. If that is not possible, use syringe and needle after proper sterilization.
  - In case the patient is agitated/not co-operating, restrain him properly with 1 or 2 assistants or wait until he calms down. It is not unusual for a broken needle leaking to a claim for compensation;
  - Confirm that it has been kept at the required temperature. If required to be reconstituted, check the diluent and whether it has got to be cooled before using.
- Always seek proper legal and medical advice before filing reply to the complainant referred to you from a consumer court.

CHAPTER NINETEEN

Examples of ADRs

Table. 19.1: ADRs of newer drugs

Drug	*ADRs*
Bosentan	Hepatotoxity
Gatifloxacin	Hypoglycemia and hyperglycemia
Nimodipine	When administered intravenously or parenterally, it can cause serious adverse events, including death.
Telithromycin	Serious liver toxicity
Clozapine	Dementia-related psychosis, paralytic ileus, hypercholesterolemia and pharmacokinetic interaction with citalopram.
Rosiglitazone	New onset and worsening diabetic macular edema, also reports of concurrent peripheral edema
Omeprazole. lansoprazole	Testicular pain, gynecomastia and impotence
Loratadine	Prostatic disorder, Glaucoma
Cyclophos-phamide	Stevens Johnson syndrome, toxic epidermal necrolysis, erythema multiforme
Losartan	Vasculitis, purpura allergic (incl. Henoch-schöenlein purpura), anaphylactic shock, anaphylactoid reaction
Raloxifene	Thromboembolic episodes
Celecoxib	GIT bleeding
HRT	Breast, endometrial cancer
Bisphos-phonates	Eye disorders
Sildenafil	Headache, flushing, abnormal vision, rhinitis, chest pain, nausea,
Zolpidem	Visual hallucinations, nausea, constipation
Olanzapine	Oculogyric crisis, retrocolitis
Carvedilol	Dizziness, blurred vision

Table 19.2: Common ADRs encountered

ADR	*Drugs*
Nightmares	Beta blockers, SSRIs, benzodiazepines, simvastatin
Anaphylactoid reaction	Vitamin K (phytomenadione)
Gingival enlargement	Cyclosporine, phenytoin and calcium channel antagonists (e.g. Nifedipine, felodipine)
Increased IOP	SSRI, steroids
Hemorrhagic cystitis	Ticarcillin
Venous thrombo-embolism	3rd generation oral contraceptive
Headache	Metronidazole, nitrates
Constipation	Antidepressants, CCBs, Iron
Diarrhoea	Iron
Gynecomastia	Phenytoin, clomiphene, isoniazid
Edema	NSAIDs, steroids, cyclosporine
Photosensitivity	Quinolones, tetracyclines, piroxicam
Bleeding episodes	Ceftriaxone, aspirin
Weight loss	SSRI, NSAIDs
Anticholinergic (dry mouth, constipation, blurring of vision)	Antidepressants, Antipsychotics
Hypokalemia	Diuretics, insulin, beta agonists
Hyperkalemia	ACE inhibitors, NSAIDs
Impairment of driving	H_1 antihistamines
Torsades de pointes	Quinidine, procainamide, dofetilide, sotalol, amiodarone erythromycin
Impotence	Thiazides, beta blockers, SSRIs, ranitidine
Hirsutism	Androgens, minoxidil
Hypotension	Alpha blockers
Flushing	Nitrates

Table 19.3: New drug interactions

Drug 1	*Drug 2*	*Effect of interaction*
Allopurinol	Azathioprine	Neutropenia
Tramadol	Antidepressants St John's wort	Serotonin syndrome Mental status changes, agitation, cyclones, hyperreflexia, shivering
Celecoxib	Warfarin, diuretics, ACE inhibitors	Renal failure
Celecoxib	Warfarin	Bleeding
Ergotamine	Erythromycin	Ergotism headache, muscle pain, numbness
Warfarin	Ciprofloxacin, norfloxacin, gatifloxacin	Bleeding
Cyclosporine	St John's wort	Rejection of transplant
Simvastatin	Nefazodone	Increased toxicity of simvastatin
Fluvoxamine Roxithro-mycin	Warfarin Warfarin	Increased effect of warfarin Bleeding
Trimetho-prim/sulpha-methoxazole	Glibenclamide	Hypoglycemia

Table 19.4: Drug induces diseases (iatrogenic diseases)

Disease	*Drug*
Parkinsonism like	Phenothiazines, metoclopramide
Cushing's habitus	Steroids
Serotonin syndrome	MAO inhibitors, SSRIs
Peptic ulcer	NSAIDs
Reye's syndrome	Aspirin
Torsades de pointes	Terfenadine
Hypo/ hyperthyroidism	Amiodarone, Lithium, OCs
Polycystic ovary syndrome Infertility	Clomiphene citrate, LH, FSH Beta blockers
Neuroleptic malignant syndrome	General anesthetics
Addison's disease	Busulfan, Ketoconazole

Table 19.5: List of banned drugs in India

1. Amidopyrine.
2. Fixed dose combinations of vitamins with anti-inflammatory agents and tranquilizers.
3. Fixed dose combinations of Atropine and Analgesic and Antipyretics.
4. Fixed dose combinations of Strychnine and Caffeine in tonics.
5. Fixed dose combinations of Yohimbine and Strychnine with Testosterone and Vitamins.
6. Fixed dose combinations of Iron with Strychnine, Arsenic and Yohimbine.
7. Fixed dose combinations of Sodium Bromide/chloral hydrate with other drugs.
8. Phenacetin.
9. Fixed dose combinations of antihistaminic with anti-diarrhoeals.
10. Fixed dose combinations of Penicillin with Sulphonamides.
11. Fixed dose combinations of Vitamins with Analgesics.
12. Fixed dose combinations of Tetracycline with Vitamin C.
13. Fixed dose combinations of Hydroxyquinoline group of drugs with any other drug except for preparations meant for external use only.
14. Fixed dose combinations of Corticosteroids with any other drug for internal use.
15. Fixed dose combinations of Chloramphenicol with any other drug for internal use.
16. Fixed dose combinations of crude Ergot preparation except those containing Ergotamine, Caffeine, analgesics, antihistamines for the treatment of migraine, headache.
17. Fixed dose combinations of Vitamins with Anti TB drugs except combination of Isoniazid with Pyridoxine Hydrochloride (Vitamin B6).
18. Penicillin skin/eye Ointment.
19. Tetracycline Liquid Oral preparations.
20. Nialamide.
21. Practolol.
22. Methapyrilene, its salts.
23. Methaqualone.
24. Oxytetracycline Liquid Oral preparations.
25. Demeclocycline Liquid Oral preparations.
26. Combination of anabolic Steroids with other drugs.
27. Fixed dose combination of Oestrogen and Progestin (other than oral contraceptives) containing per tablet Estrogen content of more than 50 mcg (equivalent to Ethinyl Estradiol) and Progestin content of more than 3 mg

Contd.

Contd.

(equivalent to Norethisterone Acetate) and all fixed dose combination injectable preparations containing synthetic Oestrogen and Progesterone.

28. Fixed dose combinations of Sedatives/ hypnotics/ anxiolytics with analgesics-antipyretics.
29. Fixed dose combinations of Pyrazinamide, other anti-tubercular drugs except combination of Pyrazinamide with Rifampicin and INH per recommended daily dose given below:

Drugs	***Minimum***	***Maximum***
Rifampicin	450 mg	600 mg
INH	300 mg	400 mg
Pyrazinamide	1000 mg	1500 mg

30. Fixed dose combination of Histamine H_2 receptor antagonists with antacids except for those combinations approved by Drugs Controller, India.
31. The patent and proprietary medicines of fixed dose combinations of essential oils with alcohol having percentage higher than 20% proof except preparations given in the Indian Pharmacopoeia.
32. All Pharmaceutical preparations containing Chloroform exceeding 0.5% w/w or v/v whichever is appropriate.
33. Fixed dose combination of Ethambutol with INH other than the following: INH Ethambutol 200 mg. 600 mg. 300 mg. 800 mg.
34. Fixed dose combination containing more than one anti-histamine.
35. Fixed dose combination of anthelmintic with cathartic/ purgative except for piperazine.
36. Fixed dose combination of Salbutamol or any other bron-chodilator with centrally acting anti-tussive and/or antihistamine.
37. Fixed dose combination of laxatives and/or anti-spasmodic drugs in enzyme preparations.
38. Fixed dose combination of Metoclopramide with systemically absorbed drugs except fixed dose combination of metoclopramide with aspirin/paracetamol.
39. Fixed dose combination of centrally acting, antitussive with antihistamine, having atropine like activity in expectorants.
40. Preparations claiming to combat cough associated with asthma containing centrally acting antitussive and/or an antihistamine.
41. Liquid oral tonic preparations containing glycerophos-phates and/or other phosphates and/or central nervous

Contd.

Contd.

system stimulant and such preparations containing alcohol more than 20% proof.

42. Fixed dose combination containing Pectin and/or Kaolin with any drug which is systemically absorbed from GI tract except for combination of Pectin and/or Kaolin with drugs not systemically absorbed.
43. Chloral Hydrate as a drug.
44. Dovers Powder I.P.
45. Dover's Powder Tablets I.P.
46. Antidiarrhoeal formulations containing Kaolin or Pectin or Attapulgite or Activated Charcoal.
47. Antidiarrhoeal formulations containing Phthalyl Sulphathiazole or Sulphaguanidine or Succinyl Sulphathiazole.
48. Antidiarrhoeal formulations containing Neomycin or Streptomycin or Dihydrostreptomycin including their respective salts or esters.
49. Liquid Oral antidiarrhoeals or any other dosage form for pediatric use containing Diphenoxylate or Atropine or Belladona including their salts or esters or metabolites Hyoscyamine or their extracts or their alkaloids.
50. Liquid Oral antidiarrhoeals or any other dosage form for pediatric use containing halogenated hydroxyquinolines.
51. Fixed dose combination of antidiarrhoeals with electrolytes.
52. Patent and Proprietary Oral Rehydration Salts other than those conforming to the following parameters:
    a. Patent and Proprietary Oral Rehydration Salts on reconstitution to one litre shall contain:- Sodium - 50 to 90 millimoles. Total osmolarity - 240 - 290 milli osmoles. Dextrose : Sodium molar ratio - Not less than 1:1 and not more than 3:1.
    b. Patent and Proprietary cereal based Oral Rehydration Salts on reconstitution to one litre shall contain : Total osmolarity—Not more than 2900 milli osmoles. Precooked rice- Equivalent to not less than 50 gm and not more than 80 gm as total replacement of dextrose.
    c. Patent and Proprietary Oral Rehydration Salts (ORS) may contain aminoacids in addition to Oral Rehydration Salt conforming to the parameters specified above and labeled with the indication for "Adult Choleratic Diarrhoea" only.
    d. Patent and Proprietary Oral Rehydration Salts shall not contain Mono or Polysaccharides or saccharin sweetening agent.

Contd.

Contd.

53.	Fixed dose combination of Oxyphenbutazone or Phenylbutazone with any other drug.
54.	Fixed dose combination of Analgin with any other drug.
55.	Fixed dose combination of dextropropoxyphene with any other drug other than anti-spasmodics and/or non-steriodal anti-inflammatory drugs (NSAIDS).
56.	Fixed dose combination of a drug, standards of which are prescribed in the Second Schedule to the said Act with an Ayurvedic, Siddha or Unani drug.
57.	Parenteral preparations containing fixed dose combination of streptomycin with penicillins.
58.	Mepacrine Hydrochloride (Quinacrine and its salts) in any dosage form for use for female sterilization or contraception.
59.	Fenfluramine and Dexfenfluramine.
60.	Fixed dose combination of haemoglobin in any form (natural or synthetic).
61.	Fixed dose combination of Pancreatin and Pancrelipase containing amylase, protease, and lipase with any other enzyme.
62.	Fixed dose combination of Vitamin B_1, Vitamin B_6 and Vitamin B_{12} for human use with effect from 01-01-2001.
63.	Fixed dose combination of haemoglobin in any form (natural or synthetic).
64.	Fixed dose combination of Pancreatin and Pancrelipase containing amylase, protease and lipase with any other enzyme.
65.	Fixed dose combination of Diazepam and Diphenhydramine Hydrochloride.
66.	Fixed dose combination of Nitrofurantoin and trimethoprim.
67.	Fixed dose combination of Phenobarbitone with any anti-asthmatic drug.
68.	Fixed dose combination of Phenobarbitone with Hyoscin and/or Hyoscyamine.
69.	Fixed dose combination of Phenobarbitone with Ergotamine and/or Belladona.
70.	Fixed dose combination of Haloperidol with any anti-cholinergic agent including Propantheline Bromide.
71.	Fixed dose combination of Nalidixic Acid with any anti-amoebic including Metronidazole.
72.	Fixed dose combination of Loperamide Hydrochloride with Furazolidone.
73.	Fixed dose combination of Cyproheptadine with Lysine or Peptone.

Contd.

Contd.

74. Fixed dose combination of Metoclopramide with other drugs except combination of Metoclopramide with Aspirin/ Paracetamol.
75. Astemizole Terfinadine.
76. Fixed dose combination of Rifampicin, Isoniazid and Pyrazinamide, except those which provide daily adult dose given below:

Drugs	*Minimum*	*Maximum*
Rifampicin	450 mg	600 mg
Isoniazid	300 mg	400 mg
Pyrazinamide	1000 mg	1500 mg

77. Phenformin for human use.
78. Rofecoxib and its formulations for human use.
79. Valdecoxib and its formulations for human use.

Table 19.6: ADRs of common drugs

Drug	*ADRs*
Pantoprazole	Headache, diarrhoea
Atorvastatin	Constipation, flatulence
Diclofenac	Hepatotoxicity
Amiodarone, chloroquine	Corneal deposits
Citalopram, nefazodone	Dry mouth, nausea
Montelukast	Headache, GIT
Nimesulide	Hepatotoxicity, chest heaviness, coronary artery insufficiency
Paroxetine	Self-harm and potentially suicidal behaviours
Tramadol	Confusion, hallucinations, dry mouth, constipation
Zopiclone	Bitter taste, dry mouth
Celecoxib	Acute neuropsychiatric events
Galantamine	Cardiac arrhythmias
Pergolide, bromocriptine	Fibrotic changes retropertoneal fibrosis
Reboxetine	Urinary symptoms
Salbutamol	Tremors
Metoclopramide	Psychiatric manifestations
Beta blockers	Sexual dysfunctions
ACE inhibitors	Dry cough
Isotretinoin	Depression

Table 19.7: Dangerous drugs these drugs have been globally discarded but are available in India

Analgin: This is a pain-killer. Reason for ban:bone marrow depression.
Droperidol: An anti-depressant. Reason for ban:irregular heartbeat.
Furazolidone: An antidiarrhoeal. Reason for ban: cancer.
Nimesulide: painkiller, fever. Reason for ban:liver failure.
Nitrofurazone: Antibacterial cream. Reason for ban:cancer.
Phenolphthalein: Laxative. Reason for ban:cancer.
Phenylpropanolamine: Cold and cough. Reason for ban:stroke.
Oxyphenbutazone: Non-steroidal anti-inflammatory drug. Reason for ban: bone marrow depression.
Piperazine: Anti-worms. Reason for ban:nerve damage.
Quiniodochlor: Anti-diarrhoeal. Reason for ban damage to eye sight.

Table 19.8: List of dubious fixed-dose combinations (FDCs) being marketed in India. But not approved in any developed country. Most of these combinations are not approved and hence illegal

Alprazolam + sertraline
Alprazolam + imipramine
Alprazolam + fluoexetine
Alprazolam + melatonin
Imipramine + diazepam
Risperidone + trihexyphenidyl
Norfloxacin + tinidazole
Norfloxacin + tinidazole + dicyclomine
Norfloxacin + tinidazole + loperamide
Norfloxacin + metronidazole
Norfloxacin + ornidazole
Ciprofloxacin + tinidazole
Ciprofloxacin + metronidazole
Ofloxacin + tinidazole
Ofloxacin + metronidazole
Ofloxacin + ornidazole
Fluconazole + tinidazole
Doxycycline + tinidazole
Tetracycline + metronidazole
Mefenamic acid + drotaverine
Nimesulide + paracetamol
Nimesulide + diclofenac
Nimesulide + dicyclomine
Nimesulide + chlorzoxazone
Nimesulide + methocarbamol
Nimesulide + camylofin
Nimesulide + serratiopeptidase
Nimesulide + tizanidine
Nimesulide + paracetamol + chlorzoxazone
Nimesulide + tizanidine + paracetamol
Rofecoxib + tizanidine
Ibuprofen + tizanidine
Diclofenac + tizanidine
Diclofenac + famotidine
Diclofenac + paracetamol + tizanidine
Diclofenac + serratiopeptidase
Diclofenac + paracetamol + serratiopeptidase
Ibuprofen + paracetamol + magnesium trisilicate
Ranitidine + dicyclomine
Sucralfate + oxethazine
Cisapride + simethicone
Cisapride + omeprazole
Mosapride + methylpolysiloxane

Table 19.9: Drugs of current interest for reporting ADRs

Bupropion	Fondaparinux
Galantamine	Gatifloxacin
Lercanidipine	Meloxicam
Mirtazapine	Moxifloxacin
Oxcarbazepine	Pioglitazone
Rivastigmine	Celecoxib
Reboxetine	Risedronate
Rosiglitazone	Sibutramine
Tegaserod	Zolpidem
Esomeprazole	Apomorphine
Aripiprazole	Ezetimibe
Nimesulide	Losarten
Levetiracetam	Tadalafil

Table 19.10: Essential drug list (2003)

A

1. Acenocoumarol
2. Acetazolamide
3. Acetyl Salicylic Acid
4. Acriflavin+Glycerin
5. Actinomycin D
6. Activated Charcoal
7. Acyclovir
8. Adenosine
9. Adrenaline Bitartrate
10. Albendazole
11. Albumin
12. Allopurinol
13. Alpha Interferon
14. Alprazolam
15. Aluminium Hydroxide + Magnesium Hydroxide
16. Amikacin
17. Aminophylline
18. Amiodarone
19. Amitriptyline
20. Amlodipine
21. Amoxicillin
22. Amphotericin B
23. Ampicillin
24. Antisnake Venom
25. Anti-D Immunoglobulin (Human)

Contd.

Contd.

26. Antitetanus Human Immunoglobin
27. Artesunate
28. Ascorbic Acid
29. Atenolol
30. Atracurium Besylate
31. Atropine Sulphate
32. Azathioprine
33. Azithromycin

B

34. B.C.G Vaccine
35. Barium Sulphate
36. Beclomethasone Dipropionate
37. Benzathine Benzylpenicillin
38. Benzoic Acid + Salicylic Acid
39. Benzoin Compound
40. Benzyl Benzoate
41. Benzylpenicillin
42. Betamethasone Dipropionate
43. Betaxolol Hydrochloride
44. Bisacodyl
45. Bleaching Powder
46. Bleomycin
47. Bretylium Tosylate
48. Bromocriptine Mesylate
49. Bupivacaine Hydrochloride
50. Busulphan

C

51. Calamine
52. Calcium Gluconate
53. Calcium Ipodate
54. Calcium salts
55. Carbamazepine
56. Carbimazole
57. Cefotaxime
58. Ceftazidime
59. Ceftriaxone
60. Cefuroxime
61. Centchroman
62. Cephalexin
63. Cetrimide
64. Chloramphenicol
65. Chlorhexidine
66. Chloroquine Phosphate
67. Chlorpheniramine Maleate

Contd.

Contd.

68. Chlorpromazine Hydrochloride
69. Chlorthalidone
70. Ciprofloxacin Hydrochloride
71. Cisplatin
72. Clarithromycin
73. Clofazimine
74. Clomiphene Citrate
75. Clomipramine Hydrochloride
76. Clonidine Hydrochloride
77. Clotrimazole
78. Cloxacillin
79. Coal Tar
80. Codeine Phosphate
81. Colchicine
82. Condoms
83. Co-Trimoxazole (Trimethoprim + Sulphamethoxazole)
84. Cryoprecipitate
85. Cyanocobalamin
86. Cyclophosphamide
87. Cyclosporine
88. Cytosine Arabinoside

D

89. D.P.T Vaccine
90. Danazol
91. Dapsone
92. Desferrioxamine Mesylate
93. Dexamethasone
94. Dexchlorpheniramine Maleate
95. Dextran-40
96. Dextran-70
97. Dextromethorphan
98. Diazepam
99. Diclofenac
100. Dicyclomine Hydrochloride
101. Didanosine
102. Diethylcarbamazine Citrate
103. Digoxin
104. Dihydroergotamine
105. Diloxanide Furoate
106. Diltiazem
107. Dimercaprol
108. Diphtheria Antitoxin
109. Dithranol
110. Dobutamine

Contd.

Contd.

111. Domperidone
112. Dopamine Hydrochloride
113. Doxapram
114. Doxorubicin
115. Doxycycline

E

116. Efavirenz
117. Enalapril Maleate
118. Erythromycin Estolate
119. Esmolol
120. Ethambutol
121. Ether, Anaesthetic
122. Ethinylestradiol + Levonorgesterol
123. Ethinylestradiol + Norethisterone
124. Ethinylestradiol
125. Ethyl Alcohol 70%
126. Ethyl Chloride
127. Etoposide

F

128. 5-Fluorouracil
129. Factor IX Complex (Coagulation Factors II, VII, IX, X)
130. Factor VIII Concentrate
131. Ferrous Salt
132. Fluconazole
133. Flucytosine
134. Flumazenil
135. Fluorescein
136. Fluoxetine Hydrochloride
137. Flutamide
138. Folic Acid
139. Folinic Acid
140. Formaldehyde IP
141. Framycetin Sulphate
142. Fresh Frozen Plasma
143. Furazolidone
144. Furosemide

G

145. Gamma Benzene Hexachloride
146. Gemcitabine Hydrochloride
147. Gentamicin
148. Gentian Violet
149. Glibenclamide
150. Glucagon
151. Glucose with Sodium Chloride

Contd.

Contd.

152. Glucose 30
153. Glutaraldehyde
154. Glycerin
155. Glyceryl Trinitrate
156. Griseofulvin

H

157. Haloperidol
158. Halothane
159. Heparin Sodium
160. Hepatitis B Vaccine
161. Homatropine
162. Hormone Releasing IUD
163. Hydrochlorothiazide
164. Hydrocortisone Sodium Succinate
165. Hydrogen Peroxide
166. Hydroxyethyl Starch (Hetastarch)
167. Hyoscine Butyl Bromide
168. Ibuprofen
169. Imipramine
170. Indinavir
171. Insulin Injection (Soluble)
172. Intermediate Acting Insulin (Lente/NPH Insulin)
173. Intraperitoneal Dialysis Solution (of approximate composition)
174. Iodine
175. Iopanoic Acid
176. Iron Dextran
177. Isoflurane
178. Isoniazid
179. Isoprenaline Hydrochloride
180. Isosorbide 5 Mononitrate/Dinitrate
181. Isoxsuprine Hydrochloride
182. Isphaghula
183. IUD containing Copper

K

184. Ketamine Hydrochloride
185. Ketoconazole

L

186. L- Asparaginase
187. Lamivudine + Zidovudine
188. Lamivudine +Nevirapine + Stavudine
189. Lamivudine
190. Levodopa+ Carbidopa
191. Levothyroxine

Contd.

Contd.

192. Lignocaine Hydrochloride + Adrenaline
193. Lignocaine Hydrochloride
194. Lignocaine
195. Lithium Carbonate
196. Local Anaesthetic, Astringent and Antiinflammatory Medicines
197. Loperamide (Contraindicated for paediatric use)
198. Losartan Potassium

M

199. Magnesium Sulphate
200. Mannitol
201. Measles Vaccine
202. Mebendazole
203. Medroxy Progesterone Acetate
204. Meglumine Iothalamate
205. Meglumine Iotroxate
206. Melphalan
207. Menadione Sodium Sulphite
208. Mercaptopurine
209. Metformin
210. Methotrexate
211. Methyl Cellulose
212. Methyl Ergometrine
213. Methyldopa
214. Methylprednisolone
215. Methylrosanilinium Chloride (Gentian Violet)
216. Methylthioninium Chloride (Methylene blue)
217. Metoclopramide
218. Metoprolol
219. Metronidazole
220. Mexiletine Hydrochloride
221. Miconazole
222. Midazolam
223. Mifepristone
224. Mitomycin-C
225. Morphine Sulphate
226. Multivitamins

N

227. N/2 Saline
228. N/5 Saline
229. Nalidixic Acid
230. Naloxone
231. Nelfinavir
232. Neomycin + Bacitracin

Contd.

Contd.

233. Neostigmine
234. Nevirapine
235. Niclosamide
236. Nicotinamide
237. Nifedipine
238. Nitrazepam
239. Nitrofurantoin
240. Nitrous Oxide
241. Norethisterone
242. Norfloxacin
243. Normal Saline
244. Nystatin

O

245. Ofloxacin
246. Omeprazole
247. Ondansetron
248. Oral Poliomyelitis Vaccine (Live Attenuated)
249. Oral Rehydration Salts
250. Oxygen
251. Oxytocin

P

252. Paclitaxel
253. Pancuronium Bromide
254. Paracetamol
255. Penicillamine
256. Pentamidine Isothionate
257. Pentazocine
258. Pethidine Hydrochloride
259. Pheniramine Maleate
260. Phenobarbitone
261. Phenylephrine
262. Phenytoin Sodium
263. Physostigmine Salicylate
264. Phytomenadione
265. Pilocarpine
266. Platelet Rich Plasma
267. Polygeline
268. Potassium Chloride
269. Potassium Permanganate
270. Povidone Iodine
271. Pralidoxime Chloride (2-PAM)
272. Praziquantel
273. Prednisolone
274. Prednisolone Acetate

Contd.

Contd.

275. Prednisolone Sodium Phosphate
276. Primaquine
277. Procainamide Hydrochloride
278. Procaine Benzylpenicillin
279. Procarbazine
280. Prochlorperazine
281. Promethazine
282. Propranolol Hydrochloride
283. Propranolol
284. Propyliodone
285. Protamine Sulphate
286. Pyrantel Pamoate
287. Pyrazinamide
288. Pyridostigmine Bromide
289. Pyridoxine
290. Pyrimethamine

Q

291. Quinidine
292. Quinine Sulphate

R

293. Rabies Immunoglobulin
294. Rabies Vaccine
295. Raloxifene
296. Ranitidine Hydrocholoride
297. Riboflavin
298. Rifampicin
299. Ringer Lactate
300. Ritonavir
301. Roxithromycin

S

302. Salbutamol Sulphate
303. Salicylic Acid
304. Saquinavir
305. Silver Nitrate
306. Silver Sulphadiazine
307. Sodium Meglumine Diatrizoate
308. Sodium Bicarbonate
309. Sodium Iothalamate
310. Sodium Nitrite
311. Sodium Nitroprusside
312. Sodium Stibogluconate
313. Sodium Thiosulphate
314. Sodium Valproate
315. Spironolactone

Contd.

Contd.

316. Stavudine
317. Streptokinase
318. Streptomycin Sulphate
319. Succinyl Choline Chloride
320. Sulfadoxine +Pyrimethamine
321. Sulfasalazine
322. Sulphacetamide Sodium
323. Sulphadiazine

T

324. Tamoxifen Citrate
325. Terazosin
326. Terbutaline Sulphate
327. Testosterone
328. Tetanus Toxoid
329. Tetracaine Hydrochloride
330. Tetracycline Hydrochloride
331. Tetracycline
332. Theophylline Compounds
333. Thiacetazone + Isoniazid
334. Thiamine
335. Thiopentone Sodium
336. Timolol Maleate
337. Tinidazole
338. Trifluoperazine
339. Trihexyphenidyl Hydrochloride
340. Trimethoprim
341. Tropicamide
342. Tuberculin, Purified Protein Derivative

U

343. Urokinase

V

344. Vancomycin Hydrochloride
345. Verapamil
346. Vinblastine Sulphate
347. Vincristine
348. Vitamin A
349. Vitamin D3 (Ergocalciferol)

W

350. Warfarin Sodium
351. Water for Injection

X

352. Xylometazoline

Z

353. Zidovudine
354. Zinc Oxide